EYE AND VISION RESEARCH DEVELOPMENTS

CENTRAL SEROUS CHORIORETINOPATHY (CSCR)

RISK FACTORS, DIAGNOSIS AND MANAGEMENT

EYE AND VISION RESEARCH DEVELOPMENTS

Additional books in this series can be found on Nova's website under the Series tab.

Additional e-books in this series can be found on Nova's website under the e-book tab.

EYE AND VISION RESEARCH DEVELOPMENTS

CENTRAL SEROUS CHORIORETINOPATHY (CSCR)

RISK FACTORS, DIAGNOSIS AND MANAGEMENT

PATRICK EVANS
EDITOR

New York

Library of Congress Cataloging-in-Publication Data

Library of Congress Control Number: 2016963449
ISBN: 978-1-53610-806-4

Published by Nova Science Publishers, Inc. † New York

CONTENTS

PREFACE

Central serous chorioretinopathy (CSCR) is an idiopathic, self-limiting retinal disease characterized by focal leakage from choroidal vessels through an altered retinal pigment epithelium (RPE) that results in limited serous detachment of the neurosensory retina. This book provides new research on the risk factors, diagnosis and treatments of CSCR.

Chapter 1 - Central serous chorioretinopathy (CSCR) is a relatively common disease that mainly affects white men aged 30 to 50 years old. It is characterized by leakage of serous fluid from choroidal vessels through the retinal pigment epithelium (RPE) causing detachment of the neurosensory retina. The pathogenesis remains unclear but recent studies suggest that CSCR may in fact represent the ocular manifestation of a systemic microvasculopathy. Although CSCR was widely considered a unilateral disease, new evidence has identified subclinical involvement in the fellow eye of patients with CSCR. Choroidal congestion, increased vascular permeability and RPE dysfunction play a key role in the formation of subretinal fluid (SRF).

Several risk factors for CSCR have been described: corticosteroid use, increased endogenous cortisol levels, type A personality, hypertension and cardiovascular disease, pregnancy, Helicobacter pylori infection, autoimmune disease, adrenergic medication use and sleep disturbances. While cases of familial CSCR have been described, the role of genetic predisposition is unclear. Recently, polymorphisms of the complement factor H were linked to the disease.

CSCR is a predominantly self-limiting disease and usually resolves spontaneously within 3 to 4 months. The patients maintain good visual acuity but often experience long-lasting colour discrimination defects and/or metamorphopsiae. However, recurrences associated with prolonged neuroretinal detachment may lead to progressive RPE atrophy, photoreceptor damage and significant visual loss. Although the incidence of the disease has a six-fold male preponderance, the chronic or steroid-related forms seem to affect both sexes equally.

Multimodal retinal imaging has revolutionised the authors' diagnostic algorithm for CSCR. Optical coherence tomography (OCT) is the gold standard for the diagnosis and follow-up of the disease whereas enhanced depth imaging OCT has allowed the visualisation of thickened choroid in patients with CSCR. Fundus autofluorescence imaging in chronic cases is valuable in identifying RPE damage. Fluorescein angiography reveals one or more leakage sites or early pinpoint hyperfluorescence, while indocyanine green angiography (ICGA) is useful in detecting choroidal neovascularisation (CNV) in chronic cases. ICGA findings include filling delays of the choroidal arteries and choriocapillaris, venous dilation, and focal hyperfluorescence of the choroid. The recently developed OCT angiography has allowed the detection of CNV related to chronic forms of the disease and has also highlighted irregular choriocapillaris blood flow patterns.

There is currently no consensus on the most suitable treatment of CSCR and the optimal time for intervention. Since the natural course of the disease often leads to spontaneous resolution, observation is the initial approach. SRF persisting for more than 4 months with a resultant deterioration of visual acuity is an indication for intervention. Suggested therapeutic modalities include laser treatment, various protocols of photodynamic therapy, anti-vascular endothelial growth factor injections, oral mineralocorticoid antagonists, oral carbonic anhydrase inhibitors, Helicobacter pylori treatment and oral rifampicin.

Exciting developments in novel imaging platforms are expected to shed light in the pathophysiology and management of this condition. Long-term, adequately powered, controlled research on the exact role of the currently available therapeutic options for the treatment of CSCR is warranted.

Chapter 2 - This chapter summarizes and critically evaluates advances in clinical management and therapy of Central Serous Chorioretinopathy (CSCR), which are mainly driven by advances in diagnosis of the disease. Following a brief historical overview, the chapter systematically reviews advances in CSCR diagnosis, namely assessment of Best Corrected Visual Acuity (BCVA), contrast sensitivity and psychophysical parameters, fluorescein and indocyanine green angiography, Optical Coherence Tomography angiography, Spectral-domain optical coherence tomography for the assessment of choroidal, retinal and macular thickness, retinal structure, neovascularization and outer retinal reflectivity, measurement of macular choroidal hemodynamics, flash and pattern ERG, and microperimetry. Furthermore, the effect of therapies on the diagnosis of CSCR are being reviewed in the context of recent advances and for concepts under clinical development, such as effects of corticosteroids as contraindicated medications, treatment with spironolactone, acetazolamide, photodynamic therapy and anti-VEGF therapies.

Chapter 3 - The pathogenesis of central serous choroidopathy (CSCR) is a complex one, in which there is a choroidal dysfunction that leads a hyperpermeability state of the choroid and a retinal pigment epithelium (RPE) detachment and leakage of fluid into the sub retinal space, affecting the posterior pole. It has been associated with high levels of corticosteroids, both endogenous and exogenous, Helicobacter pylori infections, Type-A personalities, but in the majority it has an idiopathic origin.

Two subtypes have been described, acute CSCR and chronic CSCR. It has a usually benign natural history; it resolves without treatment usually within four to six months. In the acute phases, usually a focal leakage point can be seen on both the fluorescein angiography (FA) and indocyanine-green angiography (IGA). In chronic or recurrent cases, usually there is no focal, but a diffuse area of leakage that spreads over a wider area of the posterior pole. Extra foveal focal leakage points can be and have been treated in the past with conventional laser photocoagulation to expedite the resolution of the serous detachment, but the final visual acuity (VA) is often the same as that with spontaneous healing. The way laser works is not fully understood, although it is aimed in destroying and scarring leaking vessels with a theoretical healthy RPE cell migration that takes over the pump function. Several complications have been identified with this treatment, which include scotomas, choroidal neovascularization (CNV), retinal scarring, and contrast sensitivity. Because of these reasons, this treatment is considered ideally for patients with recurrent or chronic cases, those with permanent CSCR changes in the fellow eye, or a professional need for a quick recovery by the patient. Other treatments include anti vascular endothelial growth factor agents (anti-VEGF) as well as photodynamic therapy (PDT). PDT is not exempt from developing many of the complications as conventional laser therapy, thus leading to the development of new technologies for the treatment of macular diseases, amongst which subthreshold micropulse laser therapy of the RPE has shown results comparable to those of conventional laser therapy.

Preliminary studies with the micropulse technology were with 810nm laser, although 577nm yellow laser has stood out in recent practices. In micropulse mode, laser is delivered in short pulses that allow for a cooling of the tissues in between these. Conventional laser causes a photocoagulative effect on the neurosensory retina with a surrounding area of treatment around each burn. Micropulse laser on the other hand, creates a photothermal effect that stimulates the RPE the retinal without the burn or scarring of the neurosensory retina. This reaction is only distinguished in histological and microscopical examination, but is otherwise undetectable. Yellow laser is poorly absorbed by the xanthophyll pigment mostly found on the fovea, which allows a transfoveal treatment. Few adverse effects have been reported with the use of this laser, being retinal edema and SRF the most commonly reported. Subthreshold micropulse laser therapy presents as a treatment option for those cases in which the fovea is involved.

Chapter 4 - There is no fully effective treatment for central serous chorioretinopathy, therefore investigators have proposed and explored a series of interventional alternatives. These alternatives include local and systemic oral therapy.

The pathophysiology of the disease is still not thoroughly understood and the exact role of corticosteroids is unclear. Several hypotheses have been suggested on the physiopathology of this disease. However, recent research has demonstrated the importance of glucocorticoids and mineralocorticoids. Animal models have proved influence of these hormones on choroidal permeability, leading to usage of antiglucocorticoid medications as treatment. Pilot studies have demonstrated certain efficiency clinically with improvements in visual acuity and macular morphology. Results are varied but antiglucocorticoid medication seems to be a promising alternative.

Excessive epinephrine may affect the retina through beta-adrenergic receptors on the retinal pigment epithelium. Activation of these receptors has been shown to produce a change in cyclic adenosine monophosphate concentration, affecting retinal pigment epithelium's electrical activity. Epinephrine has also been shown to induce apoptosis in retinal pigment epithelium cells *in vitro*, leading to the proposal of propranolol and other beta-blockers as alternative therapy. Results have been mixed on the use of beta-blockers making other alternatives more promising.

The choroidal vasculature has been the base of mineralocorticoid antagonist therapy such as spironolactone, eplerenone, mifepristone and ketoconazole, or the 5α-reductase inhibiting drug finasteride.

Finasteride has been used due to its antiandrogenic effects but due to its side effects could have limitations in clinical use for CSC.

Reduction of the expression of steroid receptors has also been proposed as a target with therapy through low doses of methotrexate and melatonin but further research is necessary.

Aspiring has also been used for its effects on coagulation and plasminogen activator inhibitor. Although further investigation is required it has been found to improve visual acuity.

Rifampin is one of the most widely used and investigated oral treatments. Its properties induce cytochrome P450 therefore accelerating steroid metabolism, leading to a decrease in plasma steroids. Such decrease has been demonstrated on both exogenous and endogenous steroids, driving many case report series with promising results as a therapeutic alternative.

Recent data has demonstrated correlation between Helicobacter pylori infection and CSC. Studies have used treatment against this bacillus on patients with CSC, however results have been mixed.

There are many publications with these unconventional options, nevertheless most of them are small number case series, and require longer follow up and a larger number of cases. Randomized studies need to be published in order to understand the long-term efficiency, recurrences and safety of these non-invasive alternatives.

In: Central Serous Chorioretinopathy (CSCR) ISBN: 978-1-53610-806-4
Editor: Patrick Evans

Chapter 1

AN OVERVIEW OF RISK FACTORS, DIAGNOSIS AND TREATMENT OF CENTRAL SEROUS CHORIORETINOPATHY

Andreas Katsanos[1,*], Konstantina Gorgoli[2], Vasileios Konidaris[2] and Theo Empeslidis[2]

[1]Ophthalmology Department, University of Ioannina, Ioannina, Greece
[2]Ophthalmology Department, University Hospitals of Leicester, Leicester, UK

ABSTRACT

Central serous chorioretinopathy (CSCR) is a relatively common disease that mainly affects white men aged 30 to 50 years old. It is characterized by leakage of serous fluid from choroidal vessels through the retinal pigment epithelium (RPE) causing detachment of the neurosensory retina. The pathogenesis remains unclear but recent studies suggest that CSCR may in fact represent the ocular manifestation of a systemic microvasculopathy. Although CSCR was widely considered a unilateral disease, new evidence has identified subclinical involvement in the fellow eye of patients with CSCR. Choroidal congestion, increased

[*] Corresponding author: Andreas Katsanos, Ophthalmology Department, University of Ioannina, Stavros Niarchos Avenue, 45110 Ioannina, Greece. Tel: +302651099657, e-mail: andreas.katsanos@hotmail.com.

vascular permeability and RPE dysfunction play a key role in the formation of subretinal fluid (SRF).

Several risk factors for CSCR have been described: corticosteroid use, increased endogenous cortisol levels, type A personality, hypertension and cardiovascular disease, pregnancy, Helicobacter pylori infection, autoimmune disease, adrenergic medication use and sleep disturbances. While cases of familial CSCR have been described, the role of genetic predisposition is unclear. Recently, polymorphisms of the complement factor H were linked to the disease.

CSCR is a predominantly self-limiting disease and usually resolves spontaneously within 3 to 4 months. The patients maintain good visual acuity but often experience long-lasting colour discrimination defects and/or metamorphopsiae. However, recurrences associated with prolonged neuroretinal detachment may lead to progressive RPE atrophy, photoreceptor damage and significant visual loss. Although the incidence of the disease has a six-fold male preponderance, the chronic or steroid-related forms seem to affect both sexes equally.

Multimodal retinal imaging has revolutionised our diagnostic algorithm for CSCR. Optical coherence tomography (OCT) is the gold standard for the diagnosis and follow-up of the disease whereas enhanced depth imaging OCT has allowed the visualisation of thickened choroid in patients with CSCR. Fundus autofluorescence imaging in chronic cases is valuable in identifying RPE damage. Fluorescein angiography reveals one or more leakage sites or early pinpoint hyperfluorescence, while indocyanine green angiography (ICGA) is useful in detecting choroidal neovascularisation (CNV) in chronic cases. ICGA findings include filling delays of the choroidal arteries and choriocapillaris, venous dilation, and focal hyperfluorescence of the choroid. The recently developed OCT angiography has allowed the detection of CNV related to chronic forms of the disease and has also highlighted irregular choriocapillaris blood flow patterns.

There is currently no consensus on the most suitable treatment of CSCR and the optimal time for intervention. Since the natural course of the disease often leads to spontaneous resolution, observation is the initial approach. SRF persisting for more than 4 months with a resultant deterioration of visual acuity is an indication for intervention. Suggested therapeutic modalities include laser treatment, various protocols of photodynamic therapy, anti-vascular endothelial growth factor injections, oral mineralocorticoid antagonists, oral carbonic anhydrase inhibitors, Helicobacter pylori treatment and oral rifampicin.

Exciting developments in novel imaging platforms are expected to shed light in the pathophysiology and management of this condition. Long-term, adequately powered, controlled research on the exact role of the currently available therapeutic options for the treatment of CSCR is warranted.

Keywords: central serous chorioretinopathy, CSCR, corticosteroids, OCT, mineralocorticoids, spironolactone, OCT angiography, fluorescein angiography

1. INTRODUCTION

Central serous chorioretinopathy (CSCR) was first described by Albrecht von Graefe in 1866 and was initially called "Central Recurrent Retinitis" (Von Graefe 1866). CSCR is an idiopathic, self-limiting retinal disease characterized by focal leakage from choroidal vessels through an altered retinal pigment epithelium (RPE) that results in limited serous detachment of the neurosensory retina. This chapter summarises risk factors, diagnostic approaches and treatment strategies for this common condition.

1.1. Epidemiology

CSCR is considered to be the fourth most common cause of non-surgical retinopathies after age-related macular degeneration (AMD), diabetic retinopathy and branch retinal vein occlusion (Wang et al. 2008). The prevalence of CSCR is likely to have been undervalued. Asymptomatic CSCR-related fundus changes have been observed in the fellow eye of patients with active CSCR or in eyes of relatives of CSCR patients (Weenink et al. 2001, Lehmann et al. 2015).

There is limited epidemiological evidence on the occurrence of CSCR in different populations. A population-based study in Minnesota reported an overall incidence of 5.8 cases of CSCR per 100 000 people with an approximately six-fold male preponderance (males: 9.9 per 100 000, females: 1.7 per 100 000) (Kitzmann et al. 2008). The condition mostly affects patients between 39 and 51 years old but can occur later in life especially in women (Kitzmann et al. 2008). The chronic form of the disease also seems more common in later life (Kitzmann et al. 2008). Caucasians were thought to be the ethnic group that was most frequently affected by CSCR. However, emerging epidemiological data have refuted this notion. CSCR seems to be equally common in African Americans but the visual prognosis in this ethnic group appears to be poorer (Desai et al. 2003). Compared to Caucasians, the incidence of the disease appears to be roughly 4 times higher in Asians: in a recent population-based study conducted in Taiwan (Tsai et al. 2013), CSCR had a mean annual incidence of 21 cases in 100 000 with a male/female ratio of 1.74.

1.2. Pathogenesis

The pathogenesis of CSCR still remains unclear. Choroidal congestion, increased vascular permeability and RPE dysfunction play a key role in the formation of subretinal fluid (SRF).

The term "pachychoroid" [Gr. *pachys*: thick] was introduced in order to describe a pathologic and stable increase in choroidal thickness. Pachychoroid usually is observed in eyes with central serous chorioretinopathy (CSCR) or CSCR-like features (Lehmann et al. 2015, Warrow et al. 2013, Pang & Freund 2015). A characteristic pattern of pachychoroid is the dilatation of the large choroidal vessels in Haller's layer, which results in the compression of the overlying choriocapillaris and medium-sized choroidal vessel layer (Sattler's layer). (Pang & Freund 2015)

Abnormalities of the choroidal circulation have been documented in patients with CSCR. The changes in choroidal circulation induce an increased vascular permeability probably due to stasis, ischemia or inflammation (Nicholson et al. 2013, Yannuzzi 2010). Studies focusing on Indocyanine Green Angiography (ICGA) point towards choroidal vasculopathy with lobular ischemia and areas with venous dilatation (Okushiba & Takeda 1997, Prunte & Flammer 1996, Spaide et al. 1996). Increased hydrostatic pressure within the choroidal vasculature as well as pathological vascular permeability and fragility may result in compromised RPE function and fluid accumulation underneath the retina (Yoshioka et al. 1982).

Based on major capillary changes observed with nailfold videocapillaroscopy (NVC), a recent study suggested that CSCR is associated with systemic microvasculopathy (Erol et al. 2016). NVC is a non-invasive diagnostic procedure used for the morphological assessment of nail-bed capillaries in patients with autoimmune vasculitis, microcirculation disorders, etc. (Grassi et al. 1996, Dinc et al. 2001, Cortes & Cutolo 2007, Aytekin et al. 2011) The digital microcirculation in patients with CSCR appears to be affected with significant capillary changes such as ectasias, aneurysms, micro-haemorrhages, avascular areas, tortuosity, neo-formation, bizarre, bushy or meander-shaped capillaries and extravasation (Erol et al. 2016).

Future studies and basic research are required in order to shed light upon the pathophysiology of CSCR and improve our understanding of the disease.

2. Risk Factors

Although the pathogenesis of CSCR remains unknown, a number of risk factors have been identified.

2.1. Corticosteroids

Both endogenous and exogenous steroids have been incriminated as factors associated with CSCR. It is well documented that patients under corticosteroid treatment are at risk for CSCR (Carvalho-Recchia et al. 2002; Haimovici et al. 2004; Karadimas & Bouzas 2004). The systemic administration of steroids (oral or intravenous) carries the highest risk of CSCR. Liu et al. reported that inhaled or nasal steroids precipitate CSCR at the same frequency as systemic treatment (Liu et al. 2016). Less frequently, steroids in dermatological formulations have been linked to CSCR, (Liu et al. 2016) whereas intra-articular, epidural and periocular steroids have occasionally been connected with the disease. Following organ transplantation (kidney, bone marrow and heart), high doses of steroids are administered thus increasing the incidence of CSCR (Chaine et al. 2001, Farzan et al. 2014).

Endogenous Cushing syndrome is triggered by prolonged exposure to raised levels of endogenous glucocorticoids. Approximately 5% of patients with endogenous Cushing will develop CSCR (Bouzas et al. 1993).

Steroid use is related to the occurrence, recurrence and non-resolution of CSCR. Steroid-related CSCR has rather atypical clinical features, is often bilateral and has no gender preference (Khairallah et al. 2012). A recent study corroborated the common clinical observation that steroid-induced CSCR is not dose-dependent but seems to represent an idiosyncratic response in predisposed patients (Han et al. 2014).

Many studies link glucocorticoids with changes in choroidal blood flow, increased vascular permeability and disruption of the outer blood-retina barrier at the level of RPE (Bouzas et al. 2002). They may act synergistically with endogenous circulating catecholamines in regulating choroidal circulation. High levels of glucocorticoids, either exogenous or endogenous, have been associated with CSCR. The primary cortical adrenal hormones aldosterone and cortisol bind to the mineralocorticoid and glucocorticoid receptors respectively. However, because the two receptors are structurally similar, cross-reactivity of glucocorticoids with the mineralocorticoid receptor occurs.

Zhao et al. demonstrated that mineralocorticoid receptors are expressed in the choroidal vessels and once activated, they cause vasodilation, leakage and choroidal thickening. (Zhao et al. 2011, Zhao et al. 2010) This effect can be reversed in the presence of mineralocorticoid receptor antagonism.

2.2. Psychopathology

A significant association between CSCR and type A personality has been described (Yannuzzi 1986). People with type A personality are more competitive, ambitious, impatient and aggressive. They are preoccupied with social status, accomplishment in life, and self-esteem. These people are high-achievers and find it difficult to accept failure. Their stress levels are generally high and subsequently the levels of cortisol and catecholamines are elevated, possibly increasing the risk of CSCR. Type A behaviour is linked to psychosomatic disorders with emotional distress, depression and somatization. Most patients do not describe any specific, particularly stressful life event (Conrad et al. 2007). In addition, the association between narcissistic personality and CSCR was recently suggested (Carlesimo et al. 2014). Stress associated with a type A personality has additionally been linked to sleeping disorders, gastroesophageal reflux and peptic ulcer (Eom et al. 2012, Mansuetta et al. 2004, Cotticelli et al. 2006).

2.3. Cardiovascular Disease/Hypertension

Systemic hypertension is linked to a higher risk of developing CSCR (Eom et al. 2012). Men with CSCR have an increased risk for coronary heart disease, ischemic stroke and erectile dysfunction (Chen et al. 2014, Tsai et al. 2013). It can be hypothesized that the choroidal vasculopathy in patients with CSCR represents only one part of the spectrum of a generalized vascular disorder (Daruich et al. 2015).

Long-standing or poorly controlled systemic hypertension damages small arterioles and capillaries thus affecting blood flow to the choroid via vasoconstriction, occlusion of the choriocapillaris and disruption of the RPE (Tittl et al. 1999). In addition to increased levels of endogenous catecholamines, people with type A personality frequently have systemic hypertension, thus further increasing their risk for CSCR.

2.4. Pregnancy

Pregnancy is a significant risk factor for developing CSCR and can be explained by the high levels of circulating cortisol and catecholamines in the bloodstream (Liu et al. 2016). The risk of CSCR is increased in cases of previous or concurrent pregnancy and is higher during the third trimester (Haimovici et al. 2004). Spontaneous resolution of CSCR is often observed within one month after delivery (Errera et al. 2013). Ninety-five per cent of patients have an excellent anatomical and visual prognosis, whereas the rest develop a more persistent form of the disease (Quillen et al. 1996).

2.5. Sympathetic/Parasympathetic Activity

Autonomic function is impaired in cases with CSCR. Tewari and collaborators studied both sympathetic and parasympathetic activity and reactivity (Tewari et al. 2006). Heart rate variability indicated increased sympathetic and decreased parasympathetic activity. Autonomic reactivity was found significantly lower in CSCR patients. Stressor stimuli can induce an abnormal response of the autonomous nervous system that regulates blood flow to the choroid (Tewari et al. 2006). In animal models, the long-lasting presence of high doses of epinephrine triggers RPE cell apoptosis suggesting a potential mechanism for CSCR (Sibayan et al. 2000).

2.6. Gastrointestinal Disorders

Gastroesophageal reflux, peptic ulcer and Helicobacter pylori infection were identified as risk factors for CSCR. Mansuetta et al. reported that CSCR patients were more likely to report gastroesophageal reflux or to have used oral antiacid/antireflux treatment (Mansuetta et al. 2004). The incidence of peptic ulcer and Helicobacter pylori (H. pylori) infection is significantly higher among patients with CSCR (Chen et al. 2014, Cotticelli et al. 2006, Roshani et al. 2014). In addition, the prevalence of H. pylori infection is greater in patients with diffuse retinal pigment epitheliopathy than the general population (Mauget-Faysse et al. 2002). The exact pathomechanism still remains an enigma but H. pylori is thought to be related to focal occlusive arterial disease (Mauget-Faysse et al. 2002). It has been suggested that H. pylori infection could induce CSCR through an immune-dependent mechanism of mimicry between bacterial antigens and host proteins (Giusti 2004). Another theory suggests that microbial cytotoxin could damage the vessel walls and cause dysfunction of the choroidal microcirculation (Cotticelli et al. 2006). The treatment of H. pylori was reported to have a favourable effect on the outcome of CSCR (Casella et al. 2012).

2.7. Sleep Disturbances

There are conflicting reports on the possible link between obstructive sleep apnoea syndrome (OSAS) and CSCR. In 2008 Kloos et al. reported a 22% incidence of OSAS among CSCR patients compared to 2-4% in the general population (Kloos et al. 2008). The increased occurrence of OSAS among patients with CSCR was confirmed in several other reports (Leveque et al. 2007, Yavas et al. 2014, Huon et al. 2016). In patients with OSAS, increased levels of circulating epinephrine and norepinephrine, oxidative stress, vasoconstriction or blood coagulation abnormalities could induce CSCR (Yavas et al. 2014). In a recent study, the risk of OSAS appeared to be the same for CSCR patients and healthy controls, when the two groups were matched for age, sex and body mass index (Brodie et al. 2015). The authors concluded that the previously suggested association of OSAS and CSCR might have been the result of differences in cohort characteristics.

2.8. Drug-Induced

The use of sympathomimetic medication such as pseudoephedrine, oxymetazoline, or 3,4-methylenedioxymethamphetamine has been reported to cause CSCR (Michael et al. 2003). Pseudoephedrine and oxymetazoline are ingredients often contained in nasal decongestants, whereas 3,4-methylenedioxymethamphetamine is an illicit amphetamine. Ephedra is a stimulant plant product used by athletes as a performance-enhancing drug and weight-loss supplement. It can also be found in cold remedies, as the compound has anticongestant action. CSCR has been described in patients using ephedra (Pierce & Lane 2009). Rare cases of CSCR have been documented after the use of phosphodiesterase 5 inhibitors (sildenafil, tadalafil) contained in medications for the treatment of erectile dysfunction. (Aliferis et al. 2012).

Mitogen-activated protein kinase inhibitors are commonly used for the treatment of cancer. In patients undergoing treatment with binimetinib, serous retinal detachments have been observed. The condition is usually benign and does not include any vision threatening sequelae, so discontinuing a life-prolonging medication is not advised (Weber et al. 2016).

2.9. Circadian Disturbances/Shift Work

Recently, shift work or irregular working hours have been recognized as an independent risk factor of CSCR. Whether changing shift work and irregular working hours to regular working hours would be beneficial for the course of a patient's CSCR has yet to be determined (Setrouk et al. 2016, Bousquet et al. 2016).

2.10. Genetics

The role of genetic predisposition in CSCR has not been elucidated so far. There are sporadic reports of familial CSCR but there is no clear transmission pattern or specific genotype. Weenink et al. report that half of the patients with CSCR had at least one relative with RPE atrophy or signs of previous CSCR (Weeknik et al. 2001). Besides, approximately half of relatives of patients with CSCR have choroidal thickness more than 395 μm implying that pachychoroid could be an inherited condition predisposing to CSCR (Lehmann et al. 2015).

The complement system may be involved in the pathogenesis of CSCR. In a study investigating the genomic copy number variations in the complement 4 gene (C4), the number of copies of C4B was found to be associated with CSCR. Having no copies of C4B was a risk factor for CSCR, whereas carrying 3 copies of the gene was protective against the disease (Breukink et al. 2015).

3. Clinical Presentation

CSCR is usually self-limiting and resolves spontaneously within a period of 3 months. The visual prognosis is good as most patients maintain a visual acuity of 0.2 logMAR or better. However, the disease can relapse and the recurrences may lead to progressive RPE atrophy and visual loss. CSCR is actually a term describing either of the two distinct forms of the disease: the acute and the chronic. However, recently the 'non-resolving/persistent' and the 'recurrent' forms were also introduced.

In the acute form, patients typically describe sudden onset of blurred vision, metamorphopsia, micropsia, dyschromatopsia and central scotoma. Hypermetropization can be noticed in the visual acuity test along with a decrease in contrast sensitivity (Wang et al. 2008). Clinically, the acute form is characterized by the presence of subretinal fluid (SRF) causing serous retinal detachment that can be identified with fundoscopy or optical coherence tomography (OCT). The RPE appears to have focal or multifocal alterations and occasionally small pigment epithelial detachments (PEDs). The SRF usually resolves in 3 to 4 months without any major visual sequelae (Gilbert et al. 1984, Loo et al. 2002). Most patients experience mild colour discrimination defects after the resolution of SRF (Baran et al. 2005).

The term 'non-resolving' or 'persistent' CSCR is used to describe the cases of CSCR where the SRF persists for more than 4 months from the onset of symptoms. Spectral domain OCT (SD-OCT) frequently demonstrates elongation of the photoreceptor outer segments within the area of the serous retinal detachment (Daruich et al. 2015).

'Recurrent' CSCR usually describes an episode of acute CSCR that follows a previous one in which complete resolution of the SRF had occurred. Various studies with a long period of follow up demonstrate that in 15-50% of cases the SRF recurs (Bujarborua 2001, Levine et al. 1989, Daruich et al. 2015, Ficker et al. 1988).

There is no general consensus on the optimal timing for intervention. Self-resolution is generally not expected for SRF that has persisted for a period of 6 months. Yannuzzi et al. characterized the chronic form of the disease as diffuse pigment epitheliopathy (Yannuzzi et al. 1992). The chronic form is typically characterised by widespread RPE decompensation with areas of RPE atrophy or irregular RPE detachments. The leakage sites may or may not be active and there is progressive damage in the photoreceptor outer segments. The SRF usually persists for at least 3-6 months. Patients commonly experience decreased contrast sensitivity and moderate to severe permanent visual loss (Piccolino et al. 2005).

Even though CSCR was traditionally considered a unilateral disease, evidence has revealed subclinical involvement of the fellow eye. (Gackle et al. 1998, Bujarborua et al. 2005) For example, Bujarborua et al. reported that 32% of patients with CSCR had evidence of contralateral previous CSCR lesions such as SRF, PEDs, atrophic or depigmented RPE areas and pigment clumping (Bujarborua et al. 2005).

Choroidal neovascularisation (CNV) is a complication of the chronic form of the disease. RPE decompensation and Bruch's membrane damage might precipitate the growth of CNV in longstanding cases of CSCR (Chan et al. 2003a). Various reports have documented that 4-8% of chronic CSCR cases are complicated with CNV (Bandello et al. 2001, Loo et al. 2002). In a study with Caucasian patients, the majority of cases with CSCR and CNV (27 of 41 eyes) were found to have polypoidal choroidal vasculopathy (Peiretti et al. 2015).

4. Diagnosis

4.1. Fundoscopy

All patients with CSCR should undergo careful bilateral dilated fundus examination. The characteristic fundoscopic finding of CSCR is a round, shallow area of neurosensory retina elevation with distinct margins. Typically, this area is encircled by a halo of reflected light. In persistent cases, numerous gray-white concentrations correspond to subretinal fibrin. RPE atrophy or pigment alterations can be present in one or both eyes and indicate a previous or current episode of CSCR. (Spaide et al. 1996, Haimovici et al. 2004)

4.2. Multimodal Imaging

The diagnosis and follow up of patients with CSCR is based predominantly on multimodal imaging. This section describes key aspects of imaging in CSCR using both established and newly developed techniques.

4.2.1. Spectral Domain Optical Coherence Tomography (SD-OCT)

SD-OCT is a quick, non-invasive imaging modality used both for the diagnosis and follow-up of patients with CSCR. This technology allows the detailed qualitative (and sometimes also quantitative) evaluation of morphological changes in the retinal layers and RPE. The characteristic findings in CSCR are the presence of SRF and PEDs that may (or may not) be associated to RPE leakage sites.

The development of enhanced depth imaging (EDI) OCT technology allows in-depth visualization of the choroidal vessels and measurement of the choroidal thickness. Although choroidal thickness varies and is influenced by age, sex, axial length and circadian rhythm, thickness values over 395 μm are considered pathologic (Lehmann et al. 2015). EDI-OCT confirmed that the choroid is thicker in both the affected and the fellow eye of patients with CSCR compared to healthy individuals (Imamura et al. 2009). The increase in the choroidal thickness can be attributed to the dilatation of the large choroidal vessels in the outer choroid that compress the overlying medium and small vessels located in the inner choroid. The RPE elevations correspond to areas of mechanical stress due to underlying choroidal congestion. When CSCR resolves, either spontaneously or following treatment, a gradual decrease in the subfoveal choroidal thickness is observed (Brandl et al. 2014, Kim et al. 2015).

PEDs are very commonly observed in patients with CSCR, especially in the chronic form of the disease. PEDs are usually small, multiple and located within- or outside the area with SRF. Their morphology varies from dome-shaped to irregular or wavy flat (Van Velthoven et al. 2005) (Figure 1). The former suggests a rise of the hydrostatic pressure underneath the RPE whereas the later might be due to loss of elasticity of the Bruch's membrane as a consequence of chronic RPE elevation (Daruich et al. 2015). The areas of PEDs are associated with underlying choroidopathy and vascular congestion. Focal areas of RPE hypertrophy, atrophy or small RPE rips have been documented thus indicating a general dysfunction of the RPE (Yang et al. 2013). The exclusion of underlying choroidal neovascularization (CNV) is essential especially in longstanding cases.

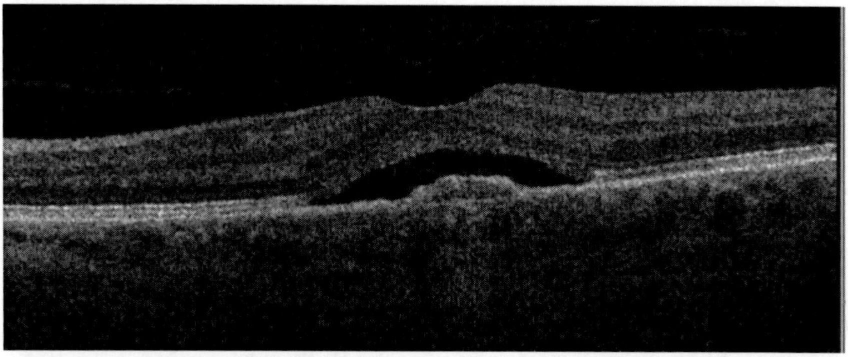

Figure 1. A case of non-resolving central serous chorioretinopathy with subretinal fluid and irregular pigment epithelial detachment.

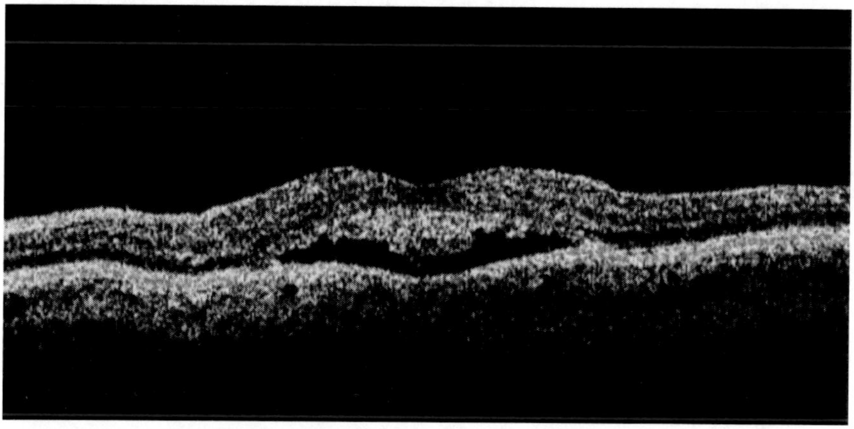

Figure 2. Persistent central serous chorioretinopathy with elongation of the photoreceptor outer segment.

The presence of SRF does not seem to affect the morphology of the retinal layers during the acute phase. However, in chronic cases, elongation of the outer segments of the photoreceptors is observed within the area of the neurosensory detachment and over the leaking site. This elongation represents a mechanical effect of abrasion of the photoreceptor outer segments from active flow through an RPE break. With time, the elongated outer photoreceptor segments accumulate and form debris-like subretinal deposits. This finding signifies a guarded visual prognosis, even after the resolution of SRF (Matsumoto et al. 2008, Yalcinbayir et al. 2014, Daruich et al. 2015) (Figure 2).

Hyper reflective dots sometimes accumulate within the retinal layers or underneath the detached retina. These are associated with chronicity, disease activity and worse visual outcome. (Yalcinbayir et al. 2014). Intraretinal cysts that can be fluctuating are usually present after several years of disease activity demonstrating a compromised activity of the RPE (Daruich et al. 2015).

4.2.2. Fundus Autofluorescence (FAF)

Fundus autofluorescence is an *in vivo* non-invasive imaging method for the metabolic mapping of lipofuscin granules that accumulate in the RPE. Since FAF evaluates the RPE integrity, the technique is an excellent method for the diagnosis and monitoring of RPE changes in CSCR.

In acute CSCR, focal areas of hypo-autofluorescence correspond to leakage sites and support the focal RPE defect hypothesis. FAF is a useful diagnostic tool to detect a focal leak in acute cases of CSCR (Eandi et al.

2005). During recurrences, the location of leakage is typically in the vicinity of the previously leaking site indicating that RPE is fragile in this area (Daruich et al. 2015).

The area of SRF accumulation appears to be hypo-autofluorescent due to masking. In enduring cases, FAF produces a patchy pattern, probably due to deposits accumulating at the elongated outer segments of the photoreceptors (Matsumoto et al. 2011). A geographic or granular decrease in FAF in the macular area is related to extensive RPE damage and poor visual acuity (Imamura et al. 2011).

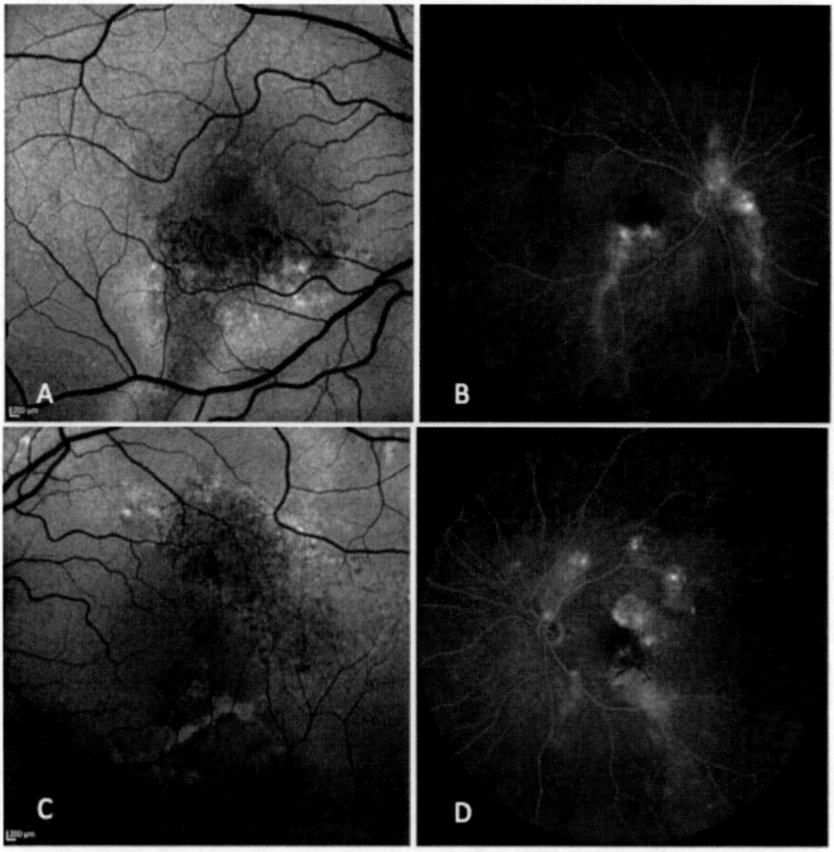

Figure 3. Bilateral gravitational tracks in a case of chronic central serous retinopathy with diffuse epitheliopathy. A: fundus autofluorescence, right eye; B: wide-field fluorescein angiography, right eye; C: fundus autofluorescence, left eye; D: wide-field fluorescein angiography, left eye.

FAF is pathognomonic in chronic cases of CSCR with the characteristic 'gravitational tracks'. These are hypo-autofluorescent patterns that arise from the macula or the optic disc and have a downward direction and a rectangular morphology. Their pathophysiology remains a mystery but it has been hypothesized that they are formed from the chronic gravity-assisted downward movement of SRF (Framme et al. 2005) (Figure 3).

Subclinical cases of CSCR or fellow eyes of patients with unilateral CSCR often have RPE changes that are detected with FAF. Their appearance varies according to the age of the lesion: new lesions appear hyper-autofluorescent whereas old lesions are mostly hypo-autofluorescent with punctate spots of increased autofluorescence (Daruich et al. 2015).

4.2.3. Fluorescein Angiography (FA)

Fluorescein angiography is not essential for the diagnosis of CSCR but is useful in confirming the diagnosis and detecting one or more leaking sites within or outside the area of neurosensory detachment. In cases of eccentric leaks, FA is used as a guide for focal laser treatment (Yannuzzi et al. 2000). In the acute phase of the disease there is usually a single leaking site. However, more than one leaking sites can be observed in some long-standing cases. In FA, the leaking sites often appear as characteristic 'pinpoints' of increasing fluorescence with time (Daruich et al. 2015). Specific angiographic patterns have been described in CSCR such as the 'ink blot' and the 'smokestack' pattern. In the 'ink blot' pattern, the leaking site appears as a distinct area of pinpoint hyperfluorescence that expands gradually to a circular area of increased fluorescence. On the contrary, in the 'smokestack' pattern the leakage has a characteristic hyperfluorescent and ascending configuration over the leaking site resembling a mushroom. Bujarborua et al. report that the smokestack form typically appears in the primary acute episode of CSCR and generally within 15 days from the onset of symptoms (Bujarborua et al. 2010).

PEDs demonstrate an early pooling of fluorescein with a persistent late hyperfluorescence (Daruich et al. 2015). Areas of RPE atrophy in subclinical cases appear as 'window defects' with increased fluorescence through defects in the RPE layer.

In the chronic forms of the disease there is generalized pigment epitheliopathy and RPE defects. In the mid phases of FA, characteristic patches of granular hyperfluorescence are observed probably due to multifocal leakage (Yannuzzi et al. 1984). The diagnosis of CNV in chronic cases can be complicated due to the coexisting features of CSCR (Figure 4).

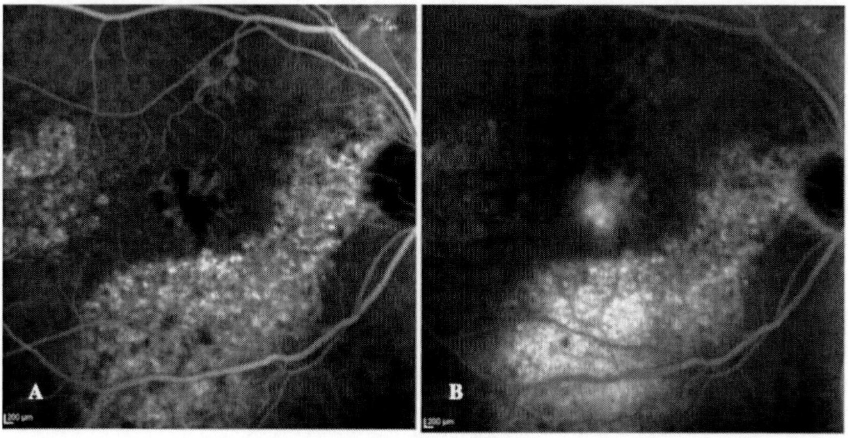

Figure 4. Early (A) and late (B) phases of fluorescein angiography in a patient with subfoveal choroidal neovascularization secondary to chronic central serous chorioretinopathy.

4.2.4. Indocyanine Green Angiography (ICGA)

ICGA is the gold standard diagnostic modality for the visualization of the deep choroidal vasculature. In CSCR, ICGA provides information about the choroidal changes associated with the disease and can distinguish CNV related to CSCR from CNV related to age-related macular degeneration (Yannuzzi 2011, Spaide et al. 1996).

ICGA demonstrates a specific pattern in cases of CSCR. In the early phase there is a delayed filling of the arteries and choriocapillaris that exhibit a decreased fluorescence (Kitaya et al. 2003). The hypofluorescence of the choriocapillaris persists until the mid and late phases. In the midphase of ICGA, a substantial dilatation of the choroidal veins is observed. There are geographic areas of hyperfluorescence with indistinct margins indicating choroidal vascular hyperpermeability (Spaide et al. 1996). During the late phase of ICGA, these hyperfluorescent areas might persist or the dye might wash-out from the centre towards the periphery forming hyperfluorescent rings (Tsujikawa et al. 2010).

Tsujikawa et al. reported that in the midphase of ICGA, 93% of eyes with active CSCR and 78% of fellow eyes demonstrated punctate hyperfluorescent spots in the macula, the peripapillary area or outside the vascular arcades. These spots seem to expand with time and it is believed to represent focal areas of vascular hyperpermeability from the inner choroidal vessels (Tsujikawa et al. 2010).

4.2.5. Optical Coherence Tomography Angiography (OCTA)

SD-OCT can be used for the study of choroidal and retinal blood vessels in a non-invasive manner using the split-spectrum amplitude decorrelation angiography (SSADA) technique. This new diagnostic modality is able to visualize capillary blood flow by detecting the movement of blood cells (Jia et al. 2012). Therefore, OCTA could be a useful tool in the investigation of choroidal blood flow in CSCR.

OCTA could not identify any leaking sites in acute CSCR (Feucht et al. 2016). The flow patterns of superficial and deep retinal plexus, outer retina and choriocapillaris do not appear to be changed. In certain cases, the choroidal blood flow appears to be affected (Feucht et al. 2016).

In chronic CSCR, OCTA has highlighted irregular flow patterns at the choriocapillaris. Focal choriocapillary hypoperfusion with surrounding hyperperfusion corresponding to ICGA abnormalities have been documented (Teussink et al. 2015).

Early data indicate that OCTA is at least as reliable as FA and ICGA to detect CNV secondary to chronic CSCR. The presence of CNV in OCTA was independent of the presence of subretinal or intraretinal fluid. CNV corresponds to the area with the irregular PEDs and it is possibly more common than previously thought (Quaranta et al. 2015, de Carlo et al. 2016). Early detection and prompt treatment of CNV could result in a better visual outcome but further research in that direction is essential.

5. Treatment

There is currently no consensus on the optimal time for intervention and the most suitable treatment algorithm of CSCR. Currently available treatment options include observation, laser treatment, various protocols of photodynamic therapy (PDT) with vcrtcrporfin (full-dose, half dose, half-fluence), anti-vascular endothelial growth factor (anti-VEGF) injections (bevacizumab, ranibizumab), oral mineralocorticoid antagonists (spironolactone, eplerenone), oral carbonic anhydrase inhibitors (acetazolamide), Helicobacter pylori eradication and oral rifampicin.

5.1. Observation/Exclusion of Risk Factors

Since CSCR is a self-limiting disease and the first episode in most patients resolves within a period of 3 to 4 months, observation should genarally be the initial appropriate approach. Unfortunately, there is no consensus on the appropriate length of the observation period. Generally, treatment is indicated in cases with SRF persisting for more than 4 months, reduced visual acuity, history of several recurrences or history of previous CSCR in the fellow eye with poor visual outcome (Nicholson et al. 2013).

The discontinuation of any corticosteroid treatment seems to be beneficial for the resolution of CSCR (Sharma et al. 2004). Patients should be informed about stopping treatment with steroids if possible. Any use of sympathomimetic drugs, signs of Cushing syndrome, pregnancy, type A personality, gastrointestinal disorders or obstructive sleep apnea should be noted and the patient should be counseled.

5.2. Laser Treatment

Focal thermal laser photocoagulation (green 514nm or yellow 580nm) is widely used in cases of CSCR as a means of sealing the RPE leaking site. Thermal laser also appears to facilitate the absorption of SRF (Robertson & Ilstrup 1983) probably by stimulating the RPE pump function of the adjacent RPE cells (Lim et al. 2011, Leaver & Williams 1979). However, thermal laser does not affect choroidal congestion and hyperpermeability (Maruko et al. 2010). Studies comparing laser treatment to observation have found that laser treatment can accelerate the resolution of SRF within a period of 8 to 10 weeks, especially when a single leaking site is documented in FA (Burumcek et al. 1997, Ficker et al. 1988, Brancato et al. 1987). On the other hand, laser therapy probably does not affect the final visual acuity and does not prevent recurrences (Burumcek et al. 1997, Ficker et al. 1988, Brancato et al. 1987). The side effects of focal laser are rare and include secondary CNV and paracentral scotoma if the treatment occurs in the vicinity of the fovea (Ficker et al. 1988, Daruich et al. 2015). Generally, laser photocoagulation is indicated in cases of acute CSCR with SRF persisting for more than 4 months due to leaking from a single site documented on FA at least 500 μm away from the fovea (Daruich et al. 2015).

Subthreshold micropulse diode laser (810 nm) has a high wavelength and (at least in principle) is absorbed exclusively by the choroid and outer retina, thus avoiding any tissue damage at the inner retinal layers (Brancato et al. 1989). This laser was advocated for the treatment of CSCR due to its superior safety profile that limits collateral tissue damage such as retinal scarring, paracentral scotomas and laser-induced CNV. The subthreshold diode laser was found beneficial for the resolution of CSCR (Bandello et al. 2003). Verma et al. randomized patients with CSCR to receive either green argon laser or subthreshold micropulse diode laser. Compared to argon laser, micropulse diode laser offered faster visual recovery, better contrast sensitivity and absence of laser-induced paracentral scotomas (Verma et al. 2004).

5.3. Photodynamic Therapy (PDT) with Verterporfin

PDT involves the intravenous administration of a photosensitizer called verterporfin, which is stimulated with a light source at 693 nm. The photosensitizer produces free radicals that cause microvascular thrombosis in neovascular tissue and choroidal vessels (Daruich et al. 2015). In CSCR, PDT with verterporfin causes choriocapillary damage and occlusion leading to blood flow stasis and decreased vascular permeability thus reducing the accumulation of fluid underneath the retina (Chan et al. 2003b, Battaglia Parodi et al. 2003).

Various reports have document that PDT can induce resolution of the SRF and significantly improve visual acuity (Yannuzzi et al. 2003, Ober et al. 2005). In one study, 94% of cases demonstrated significant reduction in choroidal permeability on ICGA following PDT (Chan et al. 2008). However, serious adverse effects and complications of PDT can occur: RPE alterations or atrophy in the treated area, choriocapillaris non-perfusion and iatrogenic CNV (Koytak et al. 2010, Lai et al. 2006). Because patients with CSCR are younger than those with AMD and usually maintain good visual acuity, their treatment settings should be different than the ones used for AMD (i.e., verterporfin 6 mg/m^2 over 10 min, laser fluence 50 J/cm^2 over 83 sec). Both lower-fluence PDT (25 J/cm^2) and half-dose PDT (3 mg/m^2) were found effective in CSCR resolution without adverse effects (Reibaldi et al. 2010, Chan et al. 2008, Stefaniotou et al. 2013). However, one-third-dose PDT (2 mg/m^2) was less effective in the reabsorption of SRF (Uetani et al. 2012). Treatment with half-dose PDT appears to facilitate more rapid resolution of the SRF, longer lasting outcome and the same safety profile compared to half-fluence PDT (Nicolo et al. 2014).

So far, there are not sufficient data to conclude which PDT protocol is superior as most studies have a short follow up. Further research is needed to evaluate the potential long-term side effects, visual outcome and recurrence rate of CSCR patients treated with different PDT protocols.

5.4. Anti Vascular Endothelial Growth Factor (Anti-VEGF) Injections

Even though VEGF levels are not increased in CSCR, anti-VEGF injections have been used in order to decrease choroidal vascular permeability (Shin & Lim 2011).

Reports comparing observation to anti-VEGF agents (bevacizumab and ranibizumab) indicate that in terms of visual acuity, treatment with anti-VEGF was not superior to observation in acute CSCR. However, a quicker resolution of the SRF was noticed, which could have a potential benefit in the preservation of photoreceptor integrity and long-term visual acuity (Park et al. 2014, Kim et al. 2013). A meta-analysis by Chung et al. failed to prove a positive effect of intravitreal bevacizumab in patients with acute or chronic CSCR (Chung et al. 2013). Furthermore, treatment with VEGF inhibitors might be unfavorable for patients with CSCR as it causes thinning of the outer layers of the retina resulting in worse visual outcome (Ozdemir & Erol 2014). On the other hand, anti-VEGF therapy is a safe and efficacious option for CNV secondary to CSCR. Chhablani et al. (2015) conducted a retrospective multicenter study with 46 eyes with CNV secondary to CSCR that received treatment with different anti-VEGF agents (bevacizumab, ranibizumab and aflibercept). With a mean number of 4.45 ± 4 injections, there was a gain in visual acuity of 1.16 ± 3.74 lines (Chhablani et al. 2015).

5.5. Oral Mineralocorticoid Antagonists

Recently, oral mineralocorticoid antagonists were introduced for the treatment of CSCR based on the pathogenetic mechanism linking aldosterone and mineralocorticoid receptors (MR) with choroidal hyperpermeability (Negi & Marmor 1984). Spironolactone, which is currently used for the treatment of systemic hypertension, is an effective but non-specific MR antagonist. In high doses, spironolactone interacts with progesterone receptors causing gynaecomastia, erectile dysfunction, decrease in libido in men and menstrual abnormalities in women (Funder 2013). On the contrary, eplerenone is a less potent but more specific MR antagonist thus having fewer hormonal side effects. Both agents can cause hyperkalemia, especially in patients with renal failure, so plasma potassium levels should be monitored regularly (Daruich et al. 2015).

Early data suggest that oral spironolactone or eplerenone at a dose of 50mg daily for 12 weeks could be useful for the treatment of CSCR as they enhance SRF reabsorption and improve visual acuity (Bousquet et al. 2013, Herold et al. 2014, Salz et al. 2015, Singh et al. 2015). Bousquet et al. conducted a prospective, randomized, double-blind, placebo-controlled crossover study with 16 patients with CSCR persisting for more than 3 months who received 50 mg/day spironolactone for 30 days. The treatment significantly reduced SRF and lead to a decrease of the subfoveal choroidal thickness (Bousquet et al. 2015). A retrospective observational study by Ghadiali et al. with a follow up of 12 months demonstrated that both spironolactone and eplerenone can decrease SRF and improve visual acuity, but the choroidal or macular thickness remains unchanged (Ghadiali et al. 2016). The response to treatment with MR antagonists is delayed in cases of persistent CSCR with gravitational tracks. Longer treatment periods are probably necessary for these patients (Daruich et al. 2016). The currently existing literature supports the use of MR antagonists in CSCR. However, randomized, prospective, long-term clinical trials are needed in order to establish their use in daily clinical practice.

5.6. Other Oral Treatments

Numerous other oral medications have been used for the treatment of CSCR. The list includes carbonic anhydrase inhibitors (acetazolamide), antibiotics (amoxicillin, metronidazole, clarithromycin), proton pump inhibitors (omeprazole) for the treatment of H. pylori, ketoconazole, rifampicin, methotrexate, melatonin, finasteride, aspirin or glucocorticoid antagonists (mifepristone). To date, the evidence on the efficacy of these medications for the treatment of CSCR is inconclusive (Nicholson et al. 2013). Further research is required to explore their potential role in the therapy of CSCR.

References

Aliferis, K; Petropoulos, IK; Farpour, B; et al. Should central serous chorioretinopathy be added to the list of ocular side effects of phosphodiesterase 5 inhibitors? *Ophthalmologica*, 2012, 227, 85-89.

Aytekin, S; Aydin, F; Akpolat, T; et al. Evaluation of nailfold capillaries in familial Mediterranean fever patients. *Clin Rheumatol*, 2011, 30, 255–257.

Bandello, F; Lanzetta, P; Furlan, F; et al. Nonvisible subthreshold MicroPulse diode laser treatment of idiopathic central serous chorioretinopathy: a pilot study. *Invest Ophthal Vis Sci*, 2003, 44, abstract 4858.

Bandello, F; Virgili, G; Lanzetta, P; et al. ICG angiography and retinal pigment epithelial decompensation. *J Fr Ophtalmol*, 2001, 24, 448–451.

Baran, NV; Gürlü, VP; Esgin, H. Long-term macular function in eyes with central serous chorioretinopathy. *Clin. Exp. Ophthalmol.*, 2005, 33, 369-372.

Battaglia Parodi, M; Da Pozzo, S; Ravalico, G. Photodynamic therapy in chronic central serous chorioretinopathy. *Retina*, 2003, 23, 235– 237.

Bousquet, E; Beydoun, T; Rothschild, PR; et al. Spironolactone for nonresolving central serous chorioretinopathy: a randomized controlled crossover study. *Retina.*, 2015, 35 2505-15.

Bousquet, E; Beydoun, T; Zhao, M; et al. Mineralocorticoid receptor antagonism in the treatment of chronic central serous chorioretinopathy: a pilot study. *Retina.*, 2013, 33(10), 2096-102.

Bousquet, E; Dhundass, M; Lehmann, M; et al. Shift Work: A Risk Factor for Central Serous Chorioretinopathy. *Am J Ophthalmol.*, 2016 May, 165, 23-8.

Bouzas, EA; Karadimas, P; Pournaras, CJ. Central serous chorioretinopathy and glucocorticoids. *Surv Ophthalmol*, 2002, 47, 431–448.

Bouzas, EA; Scott, MH; Mastorakos, G; et al. Central serous chorioretinopathy in endogenous hypercortisolism. *Arch. Ophthalmol.*, 1993, 111, 1229-1233.

Brancato, R; Pratesi, R; Leoni, G; et al. Histopathology of diode and argon laser lesions in rabbit retina. A comparative study. *Invest. Ophthalmol. Vis. Sci.*, 1989, 30, 1504-1510.

Brancato, R; Scialdone, A; Pece, A; et al. Eight-year follow-up of central serous chorioretinopathy with and without laser treatment. *Graefes Arch. Clin. Exp. Ophthalmol.*, 1987, 225, 166-168.

Brandl, C; Helbig, H; Gamulescu, MA. Choroidal thickness measurements during central serous chorioretinopathy treatment. *Int Ophthalmol.*, 2014 Feb, 34(1), 7-13.

Breukink, MB; Schellevis, RL; Boon, CJF; et al. Genomic copy number variations of the complement component C4B gene are associated with chronic central serous chorioretinopathy. *Invest Ophthalmol Vis Sci.*, 2015, 56, 5608–5613.

Brodie, FL; Charlson, ES; Aleman, TS; et al. Obstructive sleep apnea and central serous chorioretinopathy. *Retina.*, 2015, 35, 238-43.

Bujarborua, D; Chatterjee, S; Choudhury, A; et al. Fluorescein angiographic features of asymptomatic eyes in central serous chorioretinopathy. *Retina*, 2005, 25, 422-429.

Bujarborua, D; Nagpal, PN; Deka, M. Smokestack leak in central serous chorioretinopathy. *Graefes Arch. Clin. Exp. Ophthalmol.*, 2010, 248, 339-351.

Bujarborua, D. Long-term follow-up of idiopathic central serous chorioretinopathy without laser. *Acta Ophthalmol Scand*, 2001, 79, 417–421.

Burumcek, E; Mudun, A; Karacorlu, S; et al. Laser photocoagulation for persistent central serous retinopathy: results of long-term follow-up. *Ophthalmology*, 1997, 104, 616-622.

Carlesimo, SC; Piazzi, G; Leone, C; et al. Masuda's central serous chorioretinopathy (C.S.C.R.) and its somatic investment in Narcissism: our observations on new psychiatric nosography. *Clin. Ter.*, 2014, 165, 27-30.

Carvalho-Recchia, CA; Yannuzzi, LA; Negrao, S; et al. Corticosteroids and central serous chorioretinopathy. *Ophthalmology*, 2002, 109, 1834-1837.

Casella, AM; Berbel, RF; Bressanim, GL; et al. Helicobacter pylori as a potential target for the treatment of central serous chorioretinopathy. *Clinics.*, 2012, 67(9), 1047-1052.

Chaine, G; Haouat, M; Menard-Molcard, C; et al. Central serous chorioretinopathy and systemic steroid therapy. *J. Fr. Ophtalmol*, 2001, 24, 139-146.

Chan, WM; Lai, TYY; Lai, RYK; et al. Half-dose verteporfin photodynamic therapy for acute central serous chorioretinopathy: one-year results of a randomized controlled trial. *Ophthalmology*, 2008, 115, 1756-1765.

Chan, WM; Lam, DS; Lai, TY; et al. Treatment of choroidal neovascularization in central serous chorioretinopathy by photodynamic therapy with verteporfin. *Am J Ophthalmol*, 2003a, 136, 836–845.

Chan, WM; Lam, DSC; Lai, TYY; et al. Choroidal vascular remodelling in central serous chorioretinopathy after indocyanine green guided photodynamic therapy with verteporfin: a novel treatment at the primary disease level. *Br. J. Ophthalmol.*, 2003b, 87, 1453-1458.

Chen, SN; Chen, YC; Lian, I. Increased risk of coronary heart disease in male patients with central serous chorioretinopathy: results of a population-based cohort study. *Br. J. Ophthalmol.*, 2014, 98, 110-114.

Chhablani, J; Kozak, I; Pichi, F; et al. King Khaled Eye Specialist Hospital International Collaborative Retina Study Group. Outcomes of treatment of choroidal neovascularization associated with central serous chorioretinopathy with intravitreal antiangiogenic agents. *Retina.*, 2015, 35(12), 2489-97.

Chung, YR; Seo, EJ; Lew, HM; et al. Lack of positive effect of intravitreal bevacizumab in central serous chorioretinopathy: meta-analysis and review. *Eye*, 2013, 27, 1339–1346.

Conrad, R; Weber, NF; Lehnert, M; et al. Alexithymia and emotional distress in patients with central serous chorioretinopathy. *Psychosomatics*, 2007, 48, 489-495.

Cortes, S; Cutolo, M. Capillaroscopic patterns in rheumatic diseases. *Acta Rheumatol Port*, 2007, 32, 29–36.

Cotticelli, L; Borrelli, M; D'alessio, AC; et al. Central serous chorioretinopathy and Helicobacter pylori. *Eur J Ophthalmol*, 2006, 16, 4–8.

Daruich, A; Matet, A; Dirani, A; et al. Central serous chorioretinopathy: Recent findings and new physiopathology hypothesis. *Prog Retin Eye Res.*, 2015, 48, 82-118.

Daruich, A; Matet, A; Dirani, A; et al. Oral Mineralocorticoid-Receptor Antagonists: Real-Life Experience in Clinical Subtypes of Nonresolving Central Serous Chorioretinopathy With Chronic Epitheliopathy. *Transl Vis Sci Technol.*, 2016 Mar 4, 5(2), 2, eCollection 2016.

de Carlo, TE; Rosenblatt, A; Goldstein, M; et al. Vascularization of Irregular Retinal Pigment Epithelial Detachments in Chronic Central Serous Chorioretinopathy Evaluated with OCT Angiography. *Ophthalmic Surg Lasers Imaging Retina.*, 2016, 47, 128-33.

Desai, UR; Alhalel, AA; Campen, TJ; et al. Central serous chorioretinopathy in African Americans. *J Natl Med Assoc.*, 2003 95, 553-9.

Dinc, A; Melikoglu, M; Korkmaz, C; et al. Nailfold capillary abnormalities in patients with familial Mediterranean fever. *Clin Exp Rheumatol*, 2001, 19(5 Suppl 24), S42–S44.

Eandi, CM; Ober, M; Iranmanesh, R; et al. Acute central serous chorioretinopathy and fundus autofluorescence. *Retina*, 2005, 25, 989-993.

Eom, YS; Oh, J; Kim, SW; et al. Systemic factors associated with central serous chorioretinopathy in Koreans. *Korean J Ophthalmol*, 2012, 26, 260–264.

Erol, MK; Balkarli, A; Toslak, D; et al. Evaluation of nailfold videocapillaroscopy in central serous chorioretinopathy. *Graefes Arch Clin Exp Ophthalmol.*, 2016 Mar 19. [Epub ahead of print].

Errera, MH; Kohly, RP; da Cruz, L. Pregnancy-associated retinal diseases and their management. *Surv. Ophthalmol.*, 2013, 58, 127-142.

Farzan, K; Rezaei, L; Ghanbari, H; et al. Central serous chorioretinopathy following kidney transplantation. *Saudi J. Kidney Dis. Transpl.*, 2014, 25, 615-620.

Feucht, N; Maier, M; Lohmann, CP; et al. OCT Angiography Findings in Acute Central Serous Chorioretinopathy. *Ophthalmic Surg Lasers Imaging Retina.*, 2016, 47(4), 322-7.

Ficker, L; Vafidis, G; While, A; et al. Long-term follow-up of a prospective trial of argon laser photocoagulation in the treatment of central serous retinopathy. *Br. J. Ophthalmol.*, 1988, 72, 829-834.

Framme, C; Walter, A; Gabler, B; et al. Fundus autofluorescence in acute and chronic-recurrent central serous chorioretinopathy. *Acta Ophthalmol. Scand.*, 2005, 83, 161-167.

Funder, JW. Mineralocorticoid receptor antagonists: emerging roles in cardiovascular medicine. *Integr. Blood Press Control.*, 2013, 6, 129-138.

Gäckle, HC; Lang, GE; Freissler, KA; et al. [Central serous chorioretinopathy. Clinical, fluorescein angiography and demographic aspects]. *Ophthalmologe*, 1998, 95, 529-33.

Ghadiali, Q; Jung, JJ; Yu, S; et al. Central serous chorioretinopathy treated with mineralocorticoid antagonists: a one-year pilot study. *Retina.*, 2016 36, 611-8.

Gilbert, CM; Owens, SL; Smith, PD; et al. Long-term follow-up of central serous chorioretinopathy. *Br J Ophthalmol*, 1984, 68, 815–820.

Giusti, C. Association of Helicobacter pylori with central serous chorioretinopathy: hypotheses regarding pathogenesis. *Med. Hypotheses*, 2004, 63, 524-527.

Grassi, W; Core, P; Cervini, C. Increased capillary permeability in systemic sclerosis: help or hindrance? *Ann Rheum Dis*, 1996, 9, 603– 606.

Haimovici, R; Koh, S; Gagnon, DR; et al. Central Serous Chorioretinopathy Case-Control Study Group, 2004. Risk factors for central serous chorioretinopathy: a case-control study. *Ophthalmology*, 2004, 111, 244-249.

Han, JM; Hwang, JM; Kim, JS; et al. Changes in choroidal thickness after systemic administration of high-dose corticosteroids: a pilot study. *Invest. Ophthalmol. Vis. Sci.*, 2014, 55, 440-445.

Herold, TR; Prause, K; Wolf, A; et al. Spironolactone in the treatment of central serous chorioretinopathy - a case series. *Graefes Arch Clin Exp Ophthalmol.*, 2014, 252(12), 1985-91.

Huon, LK; Liu, SY; Camacho, M; et al. The association between ophthalmologic diseases and obstructive sleep apnea: *a systematic review and meta-analysis. Sleep Breath.*, 2016 May 26. [Epub ahead of print].

Imamura, Y; Fujiwara, T; Margolis, R; et al. Enhanced depth imaging optical coherence tomography of the choroid in central serous chorioretinopathy. *Retina*, 2009, 29, 1469-1473.

Imamura, Y; Fujiwara, T; Spaide, RF. Fundus autofluorescence and visual acuity in central serous chorioretinopathy. *Ophthalmology*, 2011, 118, 700-705.

Jia, Y; Tan, O; Tokayer, J; et al. Split-spectrum amplitude-decorrelation angiography with optical coherence tomography. *Opt Express.*, 2012, 20, 4710–4725.

Karadimas, P; Bouzas, EA. Glucocorticoid use represents a risk factor for central serous chorioretinopathy: a prospective, case-control study. *Graefes Arch. Clin. Exp. Ophthalmol.*, 2004, 242, 800-802.

Khairallah, M; Kahloun, R; Tugal-Tutkun, I. Central serous chorioretinopathy, corticosteroids, and uveitis. *Ocul. Immunol. Inflamm.*, 2012, 20, 76-85.

Kim, DY; Joe, SG; Yang, HS; et al. Subfoveal choroidal thickness changes in treated idiopathic central serous chorioretinopathy and their association with recurrence. *Retina*, 2015, 35, 1867-74.

Kim, M; Lee, SC; Lee, SJ. Intravitreal ranibizumab for acute central serous chorioretinopathy. *Ophthalmologica*, 2013, 229, 152-7.

Kitaya, N; Nagaoka, T; Hikichi, T; et al. Features of abnormal choroidal circulation in central serous chorioretinopathy. *Br. J. Ophthalmol.*, 2003, 87, 709-712.

Kitzmann, AS; Pulido, JS; Diehl, NN; et al. The incidence of central serous chorioretinopathy in Olmsted County, Minnesota, 1980-2002. *Ophthalmology*, 2008, 115, 169-173.

Kloos, P; Laube, I; Thoelen, A. Obstructive sleep apnea in patients with central serous chorioretinopathy. *Graefes Arch. Clin. Exp. Ophthalmol.*, 2008, 246, 1225-1228.

Koytak, A; Erol, K; Coskun, E; et al. Fluorescein angiography guided photodynamic therapy with half-dose verteporfin for chronic central serous chorioretinopathy. *Retina*, 2010, 30, 1698–1703.

Lai, TY; Chan, WM; Li, H; et al. Safety enhanced photodynamic therapy with half dose verteporfin for chronic central serous chorioretinopathy: a short term pilot study. *Br J Ophthalmol.*, 2006, 90, 869–874.

Leaver, P; Williams, C. Argon laser photocoagulation in the treatment of central serous retinopathy. *Br J Ophthalmol*, 1979, 63, 674– 677.

Lehmann, M; Bousquet, E; Beydoun, T; et al. Pachychoroid: an inherited condition? *Retina*, 2015, 35(1), 10-6.

Leveque, TK; Yu, L; Musch, DC; et al. Central serous chorioretinopathy and risk for obstructive sleep apnea. *Sleep Breath.*, 2007, 11(4), 253-7.

Levine, R; Brucker, AJ; Robinson, F. Long-term follow-up of idiopathic central serous chorioretinopathy by fluorescein angiography. *Ophthalmology*, 1989, 96, 854–859.

Lim, JW; Kang, SW; Kim, YT; et al. Comparative study of patients with central serous chorioretinopathy undergoing focal laser photocoagulation or photodynamic therapy. *Br J Ophthalmol*, 2011, 95, 514–517.

Liu, B; Deng, T; Zhang, J. Risk factors for central serous chorioretinopathy: A Systematic Review and Meta-Analysis. *Retina*, 2016, 36, 9-19.

Loo, RH; Scott, IU; Flynn, HW; Jr. et al. Factors associated with reduced visual acuity during long-term follow-up of patients with idiopathic central serous chorioretinopathy. *Retina*, 2002, 22, 19–24.

Mansuetta, CC; Mason, JO; Swanner, J; et al. An association between central serous chorioretinopathy and gastroesophageal reflux disease. *Am J Ophthalmol*, 2004, 137, 1096–1100.

Maruko, I; Iida, T; Sugano, Y; et al. Subfoveal choroidal thickness after treatment of central serous chorioretinopathy. *Ophthalmology*, 2010, 117, 1792-1799.

Matsumoto, H; Kishi, S; Otani, T; et al. Elongation of photoreceptor outer segment in central serous chorioretinopathy. *Am. J. Ophthalmol.*, 2008, 145, 162-168.

Matsumoto, H; Kishi, S; Sato, T; et al. Fundus autofluorescence of elongated photoreceptor outer segments in central serous chorioretinopathy. *Am. J. Ophthalmol.*, 2011, 151, 617-623.e1.

Mauget-Faÿsse, M; Kodjikian, L; Quaranta, M; et al. [Helicobacter pylori in central serous chorioretinopathy and diffuse retinal epitheliopathy. Results of the first prospective pilot study]. *J Fr Ophtalmol.*, 2002, 25, 1021-5.

Michael, JC; Pak, J; Pulido, J; et al. Central serous chorioretinopathy associated with administration of sympathomimetic agents. *Am. J. Ophthalmol.*, 2003, 136, 182-185.

Negi, A; Marmor, MF. Experimental serous retinal detachment and focal pigment epithelial damage. *Arch Ophthalmol*, 1984, 102, 445– 449.

Nicholson, B; Noble, J; Forooghian, F; et al. Central serous chorioretinopathy: update on pathophysiology and treatment. *Surv. Ophthalmol.*, 2013, 58, 103-126.

Nicolo, M; Eandi, CM; Alovisi, C; et al. Half-fluence versus half-dose photodynamic therapy in chronic central serous chorioretinopathy. *Am. J. Ophthalmol.*, 2014, 157, 1033-1037.

Ober, MD; Yannuzzi, LA; Do, DV; et al. Photodynamic therapy for focal retinal pigment epithelial leaks secondary to central serous chorioretinopathy. *Ophthalmology*, 2005, 112, 2088–2094.

Okushiba, U; Takeda, M. Study of choroidal vascular lesions in central serous chorioretinopathy using indocyanine green angiography. *Nihon Ganka Gakkai Zasshi*, 1997, 101, 74–82.

Ozdemir, O; Erol, MK. Morphologic changes and visual outcomes in resolved central serous chorioretinopathy treated with ranibizumab. *Cutan Ocul Toxicol.*, 2014, 33, 122-6.

Pang, CE; Freund, KB. Pachychoroid neovasculopathy. *Retina.*, 2015, 35(1), 1-9.

Park, SU; Lee, SJ; Kim, M. Intravitreal anti-vascular endothelial growth factor versus observation in acute central serous chorioretinopathy: one-year results. *Korean J Ophthalmol.*, 2014, 28, 306-13.

Peiretti, E; Ferrara, DC; Caminiti, G; et al. Choroidal neovascularization in Caucasian patients with longstanding central serous chorioretinopathy. *Retina*, 2015, 35(7), 1360-7.

Piccolino, FC; de la Longrais, RR; Ravera, G; et al. The foveal photoreceptor layer and visual acuity loss in central serous chorioretinopathy. *Am. J. Ophthalmol.*, 2005, 139, 87-99.

Pierce, KK; Lane, RG. Central serous chorioretinopathy associated with the use of ephedra. *Retin Cases Brief. Rep.*, 2009, 3, 376-378.

Prunte, C; Flammer, J. Choroidal capillary and venous congestion in central serous chorioretinopathy. *Am J Ophthalmol*, 1996, 121, 26–34.

Quaranta-El Maftouhi, M; El Maftouhi, A; Eandi, CM. Chronic central serous chorioretinopathy imaged by optical coherence tomographic angiography. *Am J Ophthalmol.*, 2015, 160, 581-587.

Quillen, DA; Gass, DM; Brod, RD; et al. Central serous chorioretinopathy in women. *Ophthalmology.*, 1996, 103, 72-9.

Reibaldi, M; Cardascia, N; Longo, A; et al. Standard-fluence versus low-fluence photodynamic therapy in chronic central serous chorioretinopathy: a nonrandomized clinical trial. *Am. J. Ophthalmol.*, 2010, 149, 307, e2-315.e2.

Robertson, DM; Ilstrup, D. Direct, indirect, and sham laser photocoagulation in the management of central serous chorioretinopathy. *Am. J. Ophthalmol.*, 1983, 95, 457-466.

Roshani, M; Ahangar Davoodi, N; Seyed Majidi, MR; et al. Association of Helicobacter pylori with central serous chorioretinopathy in Iranian patients. *Gastroenterol Hepatol Bed Bench*, 2014, 7(1), 63-67.

Salz, DA; Pitcher, JD; 3rd, Hsu, J; et al. Oral eplerenone for treatment of chronic central serous chorioretinopathy: a case series. *Ophthalmic Surg Lasers Imaging Retina.*, 2015 46, 439-44.

Setrouk, E; Hubault, B; Vankemmel, F; et al. Circadian disturbance and idiopathic central serous chorioretinopathy. *Graefes Arch Clin Exp Ophthalmol.*, 2016 May 21. [Epub ahead of print].

Sharma, T; Shah, N; Rao, M; et al. Visual outcome after discontinuation of corticosteroids in atypical severe central serous chorioretinopathy. *Ophthalmology*, 2004, 111, 1708-1714.

Shin, MC; Lim, JW. Concentration of cytokines in the aqueous humor of patients with central serous chorioretinopathy. *Retina*, 2011, 31, 1937–1943.

Sibayan, SA; Kobuch, K; Spiegel, D; et al. Epinephrine, but not dexamethasone, induces apoptosis in retinal pigment epithelium cells *in vitro*: possible implications on the pathogenesis of central serous chorioretinopathy. *Graefes Arch. Clin. Exp. Ophthalmol.*, 2000, 238, 515-519.

Singh, RP; Sears, JE; Bedi, R; et al. Oral eplerenone for the management of chronic central serous chorioretinopathy. *Int J Ophthalmol.*, 2015, 8, 310-4.

Spaide, RF; Hall, L; Haas, A; et al. Indocyanine green videoangiography of older patients with central serous chorioretinopathy. *Retina*, 1996, 16, 203-213.

Stefaniotou, M; Vourda, E; Katsanos, A; et al. Multifocal central serous chorioretinopathy associated with steroids in a patient with myasthenia gravis. *Case Rep Ophthalmol.*, 2013 Jun 1, 4(2), 1-6.

Teussink, MM; Breukink, MB; van Grinsven, MJJP; et al. OCT angiography compared to fluorescein and indocyanine green angiography in chronic central serous chorioretinopathy. *Invest Ophthalmol Vis Sci.*, 2015, 56, 5229–5237.

Tewari, HK; Gadia, R; Kumar, D; et al. Sympathetic-parasympathetic activity and reactivity in central serous chorioretinopathy: a case-control study. Invest. *Ophthalmol. Vis. Sci.*, 2006, 47, 3474-3478.

Tittl, MK; Spaide, RF; Wong, D; et al. Systemic findings associated with central serous chorioretinopathy. *Am J Ophthalmol*, 1999, 128, 63–68.

Tsai, DC; Chen, SJ; Huang, CC; et al. Epidemiology of idiopathic central serous chorioretinopathy in Taiwan, 2001-2006: a population-based study. *PloS One.*, 2013 Jun 24, 8(6), e66858.

Tsujikawa, A; Ojima, Y; Yamashiro, K; et al. Punctate hyperfluorescent spots associated with central serous chorioretinopathy as seen on indocyanine green angiography. *Retina*, 2010, 30, 801-809.

Uetani, R; Ito, Y; Oiwa, K; et al. Half-dose vs one-third-dose photodynamic therapy for chronic central serous chorioretinopathy. *Eye*, 2012, 26, 640-649.

Van Velthoven, ME; Verbraak, FD; Garcia, PM; et al. Evaluation of central serous retinopathy with en face optical coherence tomography. *Br J Ophthalmol.*, 2005, 89, 1483-8.

Verma, L; Sinha, R; Venkatesh, P; et al. Comparative evaluation of diode laser versus argon laser photocoagulation in patients with central serous retinopathy: a pilot, randomized controlled trial [ISRCTN84128484]. *BMC Ophthalmol.*, 2004, 4, 15.

Von, Graefe. Ueber central recidievendre Retinitis. *Graefe Arch Clin Exp. Ophthalmol.*, 1866, 12, 211-15.

Wang, M; Munch, IC; Hasler, PW; et al. Central serous chorioretinopathy. *Acta Ophthalmol.*, 2008, 86, 126-145.

Warrow, DJ; Hoang, QV; Freund, KB. Pachychoroid pigment epitheliopathy. *Retina.*, 2013, 33, 1659–72.

Weber, ML; Liang, MC; Flaherty, KT; et al. Subretinal Fluid Associated With MEK Inhibitor Use in the Treatment of Systemic Cancer JAMA Ophthalmol., 2016 Jun 16. [Epub ahead of print].

Weenink, AC; Borsje, RA; Oosterhuis, JA. Familial chronic central serous chorioretinopathy. *Ophthalmologica*, 2001, 215, 183-7.

Yalcinbayir, O; Gelisken, O; Akova-Budak, B; et al. Correlation of spectral domain optical coherence tomography findings and visual acuity in central serous chorioretinopathy. *Retina*, 2014, 34, 705-712.

Yang, L; Jonas, JB; Wei, W. Optical coherence tomography-assisted enhanced depth imaging of central serous chorioretinopathy. *Invest. Ophthalmol. Vis. Sci.*, 2013, 54, 4659-4665.

Yannuzzi, LA; Freund, KB; Goldbaum, M; et al. Polypoidal choroidal vasculopathy masquerading as central serous chorioretinopathy. *Ophthalmology*, 2000, 107, 767-777.

Yannuzzi, LA; Shakin, JL; Fisher, YL; et al. Peripheral retinal detachments and retinal pigment epithelial atrophic tracts secondary to central serous pigment epitheliopathy. *Ophthalmology*, 1984, 91, 1554-1572.

Yannuzzi, LA; Slakter, JS; Gross, NE; et al. Indocyanine green angiography-guided photodynamic therapy for treatment of chronic central serous chorioretinopathy: a pilot study. *Retina*, 2003, 23, 288–298.

Yannuzzi, LA; Slakter, JS; Kaufman, SR; et al. Laser treatment of diffuse retinal pigment epitheliopathy. *Eur. J. Ophthalmol.*, 1992, 2, 103-114.

Yannuzzi, LA. Central serous chorioretinopathy: a personal perspective. *Am J Ophthalmol*, 2010, 149, 361–363.

Yannuzzi, LA. Indocyanine green angiography: a perspective on use in the clinical setting. *Am. J. Ophthalmol.*, 2011, 151, 745, e1-751.e1.

Yannuzzi, LA. Type A behaviour and central serous chorioretinopathy. *Trans. Am. Ophthalmol. Soc.*, 1986, 84, 799-845.

Yavaş, GF; Küsbeci, T; Kaşikci, M; et al. Obstructive sleep apnea in patients with central serous chorioretinopathy. *Curr Eye Res.*, 2014, 39, 88-92.

Yoshioka, H; Katsume, Y; Akune, H. Experimental central serous chorioretinopathy in monkey eyes: fluorescein angiographic findings. *Ophthalmologica.*, 1982, 185(3), 168-78.

Zhao, M; Bousquet, E; Valamanesh, et al. Differential regulations of AQP4 and Kir4.1 by triamcinolone acetonide and dexamethasone in the healthy and inflamed retina. *Invest Ophthalmol Vis Sci*, 2011, 52, 6340–6347.

Zhao, M; Valamanesh, F; Celerier, I; et al. The neuroretina is a novel mineralocorticoid target: aldosterone up-regulates ion and water channels in Müller glial cells. *FASEB J*, 2010, 24, 3405–3415.

Reviewed by: Dr Panagiotis Nanos, MD
Ophthalmology Clinic of the Democritus University of Thrace, Alexandroupolis, Greece

In: Central Serous Chorioretinopathy (CSCR) ISBN: 978-1-53610-806-4
Editor: Patrick Evans

Chapter 2

NOVEL DIAGNOSTIC MODALITIES AS THE BASIS FOR SUCCESSFUL CLINICAL MANAGEMENT AND THERAPY OF CENTRAL SEROUS CHORIORETINOPATHY (CSCR)

Brian F. Jimenez*[1*]*, Sharon L. Sabapathypillai*[1*]*,
Nancy Kunjukunju*[1]*, R. Scott Duncan*[1]*,
Michael A. Cassell*[1]*, Abraham Poulose*[1]*,
Nelson R. Sabates*[1]*, Felix N. Sabates*[1]
***and Peter Koulen*[1,2+]**

[1]Vision Research Center, Department of Ophthalmology and
[2]Department of Basic Medical Science,
University of Missouri – Kansas City,
School of Medicine, Kansas City, MO, US

ABSTRACT

This chapter summarizes and critically evaluates advances in clinical management and therapy of Central Serous Chorioretinopathy (CSCR), which are mainly driven by advances in diagnosis of the disease. Following a brief historical overview, the chapter systematically reviews

---

* Contributed equally, listed in alphabetical order.
+ Corresponding Author: Peter Koulen; Email: koulenp@umkc.edu

advances in CSCR diagnosis, namely assessment of Best Corrected Visual Acuity (BCVA), contrast sensitivity and psychophysical parameters, fluorescein and indocyanine green angiography, Optical Coherence Tomography angiography, Spectral-domain optical coherence tomography for the assessment of choroidal, retinal and macular thickness, retinal structure, neovascularization and outer retinal reflectivity, measurement of macular choroidal hemodynamics, flash and pattern ERG, and microperimetry. Furthermore, the effect of therapies on the diagnosis of CSCR are being reviewed in the context of recent advances and for concepts under clinical development, such as effects of corticosteroids as contraindicated medications, treatment with spironolactone, acetazolamide, photodynamic therapy and anti-VEGF therapies.

Keywords: acetazolamide, angiography, central serous chorioretinopathy, choroid, choroidal hemodynamics, corticosteroid, electroretinography, ERG, macula, microperimetry, neovascularization, optical coherence tomography, photodynamic therapy, retina, spectral-domain optical coherence tomography, spironolactone, VEGF, vascular endothelial growth factor

INTRODUCTION

Central Serous Chorioretinopathy (CSCR), an idiopathic condition affecting the retina-retinal pigment epithelium interface, is clinically manifested as a detachment of the sensory retina that can present either unilaterally or bilaterally. Symptoms include blurred vision, metamorphopsia, and a perceived floating dark spot in the center of the visual field with ophthalmic signs ranging from mono- to pauci-focal retinal pigment epithelium (RPE) lesions with an elevation of the sensory retina with clear choroidal fluid [1]. The condition is non–inflammatory in nature affecting the function of the retina and RPE, often with increased vascular permeability throughout the choriocapillaris and buildup of sub-retinal fluid in conjunction with pigment epithelial detachment (PED) [2-4].

Dysfunction of RPE cells is one of the presumptive causes of the condition as these cells create a physiological barrier between the retina and the choroid, commonly referred to as the blood retina barrier, which is the anatomical and physiological basis of an immune-privileged space [2]. Dysfunction of the choroidal circulation is another factor that may contribute to the genesis of CSCR [3]. Increased vascular permeability leads to fluid leakage and subsequent accumulation causing distortion of the retinal structure and loss of anatomical and physiological integrity.

Retinal detachment from the choroid can distort vision or lead to loss of vision depending on the extent of the condition. In chronic cases, vision loss can be irreversible due to the extensive degree of RPE damage that causes cell death in the retina [3]. CSCR patients have increased retinal blood vessel diameters and, as such, this increased vascularization possibly contributes to an increase in choroidal thickness potentially causing the formation of subretinal fluid & PED [5].

A range of visual system conditions have been associated with a lower incidence of CSCR including emmetropia, hypermetropia, and astigmatism [6]. Since there is a potential to misdiagnose CSCR as similarly presenting, yet unrelated diseases, such as posterior uveitis or Acute Vogt-Koyanagi-Harada Disease, resulting treatment decisions can have an additional impact on disease severity [7]. In patients diagnosed with uveitis, the use of corticosteroids to treat inflammation is common, however, CSCR patients do not have elevated levels of cytokines or other inflammatory factors [8]. Unfortunately, misdiagnosis of CSCR can result in administration of certain therapies, such as steroids, which potentially worsen symptoms and outcomes [7].

The use of diagnostic imaging methods of the retina, such as fluorescein angiography, indocyanine green angiography, and optical coherence tomography, lead to improved identification of CSCR with fewer misdiagnoses and more successful treatment [3]. The most common treatment modalities, such as conventional laser therapy, photodynamic therapy (PDT), and intravitreal injection of biologicals targeting neovascularization [4], are not without side effects.

In conventional laser therapy, the induction of thermal burns effectively reduces sub-retinal fluid, but potential complications include scotomas, loss of contrast sensitivity, foveal damage, and choroidal neovascularization [4]. Similarly, PDT, while an effective treatment method, can lead to RPE atrophy and choroid ischemia [4].

Research into the CSCR disease causing process has been driven primarily by clinical evidence. The most common patient population affected by CSCR are young adults between the ages of twenty-five to fifty years, mainly presenting in men with type A personalities [9]. CSCR has been diagnosed in postmenopausal women receiving exogenous testosterone for symptoms of menopause and libido loss [10]. In women below the age of 50, CSCR presents with sub retinal precipitates, shorter lasting blurred vision and is often a one-time occurrence [11]. In women above the age of 50, however, CSCR is diagnosed with a concomitant PED and takes longer to recover [11]. In addition, genetic factors may predispose individuals to develop CSCR, with fifty-two percent of twenty-seven families studied having one or more relatives affected with CSCR [12]. Ethnic predisposition for the development of CSCR, although noted in case reports, is inconclusive [13].

In order to accurately assess CSCR, expand research into its causes and treatment and monitor therapy outcomes, the care of CSCR patients requires improved diagnostic techniques.

Assessment of Best Corrected Visual Acuity (BCVA), Contrast Sensitivity and Psychophysical Parameters

CSCR is most commonly associated with blurred vision which can eventually lead to vision loss following reoccurrences [14]. CSCR can be diagnosed by measuring visual acuity, light sensitivity and psychophysical parameters. In the study by Fujita and colleagues, seven eyes of patients with CSCR and six control eyes were examined [15]. Patients with CSCR performed more poorly at low luminance than normal controls [15] and the authors concluded that low luminance visual acuity might help diagnose patients with CSCR [15]. CSCR patients commonly present with retinal atrophy after a long duration of the disease. Wang and colleagues suggested that severe reduction of foveal thickness and multifocal retinal pigment abnormalities are only seen after ten years of disease duration and that retinal attenuation was seen after a four-month period of symptoms with CSCR [16]. At the same time, consideration of parameters measuring optical quality is also indicated in CSCR patients as the CSCR disease process can affect these negatively and increase intraocular scattering [17].

In addition to the assessment of best corrected visual acuity (BCVA), it is important to consider contrast sensitivity and psychophysical parameters in the diagnosis of CSCR. In a recent study, history and contrast sensitivity were determined to play a key role in the correct diagnosis of CSCR at different stages and may be more important in the assessment of visual acuity than BCVA [18]. Similarly, contrast sensitivity and psycho-visual assessments appear to identify macular changes more precisely than commonly used examination methods [19]. Psycho-visual examination of CSCR patients also reveals deterioration in color discrimination while contrast sensitivity tests can show undetected anatomic and functional loss even if patients present with a mild form of CSCR [20]. Though CSCR is primarily associated with blurred vision, ophthalmologists can use contrast sensitivity and psychophysical parameters to diagnose CSCR.

Fluorescein and Indocyanine Green Angiography

Since CSCR is a disease of the retinal pigment epithelium and choroidal blood vessels, it is considered to be a type of retinal pigment epitheliopathy [21]. This condition involves atrophy of the epithelium, hyper-permeability of the blood vessels, and photoreceptor atrophy [21]. Fluorescein angiography (FA) and indocyanine green angiography (ICGA) are helpful techniques to pinpoint affected areas to diagnose CSCR. ICGA allows for assessment of barrier function and metabolic status of the epithelium [21] and it detects choroidal changes in patients who present with chronic symptoms [22]. In seventeen CSCR patients, ICGA revealed common zones of increased choroidal vessel permeability and was useful for detecting other abnormalities in the choroid such as filling delay, venous dilation, and sub-retinal leakage [23].

In addition to ICGA, FA is commonly used in the diagnosis of CSCR and for the assessment of sub retinal fluid. Using ICGA, Pang and colleagues detected dilated blood vessels and hyper-permeability in twenty-four CSCR eyes that correlated with distorted FA wide-field tests. Furthermore, the authors concluded that FA and ICGA can help spot CSCR in an image identifying peripheral areas of damage and choroidal hyper-permeability [24] thus enabling objective monitoring for disease progression and therapy outcomes in CSCR. ICGA is also used with dye-enhanced micro-pulsed diode laser photocoagulation for treatment of CSCR [25] as study participants receiving such a treatment had improved visual acuity and decreased PED size [25]. As such, ICGA enhanced subthreshold micro-pulsed diode laser photocoagulation might represent an effective treatment of CSCR. In summary, FA and ICGA are not only valuable diagnostic tools but may also aid in the treatment of CSCR.

Optical Coherence Tomography Angiography

One major hallmark of CSCR is irregular choroidal blood flow [26]. The choroid is a vital for the function of the retina and optical coherence tomography (OCT) angiography has led to a wider range of imaging modalities for the choroid and its anatomy [27]. OCT images can be used to identify post-ischemic attenuation and atrophy of the retina [26] and it is being used frequently to diagnose and evaluate CSCR. Teussink and colleagues studied flow abnormalities and sub retinal fluid in eighteen eyes with chronic CSCR using OCT [26]. Their findings using OCT revealed that an abnormal choriocapillaris had reduced blood flow in certain areas and that the irregular choriocapillary flow patterns on OCT angiography may indicate areas of retinal fluid leakage in CSCR [27].

OCT angiography also allows clinicians to calculate the amount of serous detachment, track the resolution of sub-retinal fluid accumulation [28] and detect choroidal neovascularization [29]. Choroidal neovascularization corresponds with subtle RPE detachment detected with OCT angiography in patients with CSCR [29]. Iida and colleagues describe areas of low reflectivity in the OCT as an infiltrate that accumulates in the sub-retinal space and outer retina in patients with CSCR [30]. Technological advances driving retinal imaging such as OCT and related image processing [31], are critical for improved evaluation and diagnosis of CSCR.

Spectral-Domain Optical Coherence Tomography

Spectral-domain optical coherence tomography (SD-OCT) is a diagnostic test enabling imaging of the vitreous, retina, and choroid [32]. In SD-OCT, hypo-reflectivity of the choroid and structural changes measured in the RPE correlate with visual acuity deficiencies in patients with CSCR [32], potentially reducing the need for more invasive testing [33] facilitating the detection of polypoidal choroid vasculopathy versus choroidal neovascularization [33]. With the use of SD-OCT, changes in both foveal thickness, which may precede decreased visual performance, and buildup of sub-retinal fluid can be quantified [34, 35]. Correlating visual acuity with measures of foveal atrophy and the extent of sub-retinal fluid is critical for the care of CSCR patients [36]. Along with blurred vision occurring in CSCR patients, most patients also lose sensitivity in the macular region of the retina [36].

SD-OCT is becoming increasingly important in the visualization and assessment of altered outer retinal reflectivity capturing the photoreceptor layer and sub-retinal fluid in fundus images [37]. Outer retinal reflectivity using SD-OCT can be directly associated with cone density and photoreceptor density [38]. SD-OCT contributes to a comprehensive assessment of the CSCR disease phenotype potentially leading to improved diagnostic and treatment paradigms.

Laser Speckle Flowgraphy and Measurement of Macular Choroidal Hemodynamics

A key feature in the diagnosis and evaluation of CSCR is the accurate determination of choroidal blood flow velocity in the macula. Saito et al. found that macular choroidal blood flow velocity was directly proportional to CSCR disease severity [39]. As such, when CSCR symptoms decreased, choroidal blood flow velocity in the macula decreased as well [39]. Laser speckle flowgraphy identified that CSCR disease severity was associated with altered blood flow due to increased vascular resistance, which may potentially contribute to CSCR pathogenesis [40]. Laser speckle flowgraphy specifically allows for detection of the blood flow to the optic nerve head, choroid, retina, and iris [41].

FA and ICGA combined with confocal scanning laser ophthalmoscopy and laser Doppler flowmetry enables the quantitative observation of the change in choroidal circulation. For example, decreased choroidal blood flow is associated with hypo-fluorescent areas observed in ICGAs [42]. Laser speckle flowgraphy is a versatile tool for the diagnosis and monitoring of disease progression of CSCR, but also has limitations. Laser speckle flowgraphy measurements are affected by the size of the pupil and require the use of an argon laser in order to achieve separate measurements for choroidal and retinal blood flow [43]. Despite these limitations, laser speckle flowgraphy is an additional and useful tool to determine macular choroidal blood flow velocity for the diagnosis and continued monitoring of CSCR.

ELECTRORETINOGRAPHY

Vision impairment or vision loss are major symptoms in CSCR patients. In this context, electroretinography aids in detecting recurrent loss of function in the retina of patients with CSCR [43]. A standard flash or Ganzfeld electroretinogram (ERG) is useful in determining if visual impairment in CSCR is limited to the macula, since deficiencies in the P50 component of the pattern ERG indicates visual acuity and visual impairment [44]. Multifocal ERGs provide significant diagnostic information for the evaluation of CSCR disease severity when combined with OCT [45]. Retinal responses of CSCR eyes measured with multifocal ERG before treatment were significantly reduced by approximately 50% when compared to normal eyes. However, after resolution of CSCR multifocal ERG were still about 30% lower than in controls [45].

MICROPERIMETRY

In CSCR, microperimetry measurements indicate that the macula is usually more affected than the periphery; patients present with a loss of sensitivity in the central and para-central regions and possible central vision loss, while fixation in affected eyes remained stable and central [46]. These areas of central sensitivity loss measured with microperimetry were also positively correlated with changes in central fundus autofluorescence. Autofluorescence is absent in areas of scotoma, and some autofluorescence can be detected in central areas along with a loss of sensitivity. [47]. Among the diagnostic modalities used for the care of CSCR, microperimetry facilitates the study of the macula and diagnosis of CSCR, but is also useful to correlate changes in retinal sensitivity with changes in retinal structure, especially in combination with other diagnostic tools [48, 49] and by using established normative databases [50].

CSCR patients typically display decreased retinal sensitivity within the foveal center zone, which correlates to a change in retinal sensitivity and central retinal thickness [48, 49]. In addition to detecting the association between retinal sensitivity and retinal structural changes when combined with OCT, microperimetry can also be used effectively in determining functional effects of persistent sub-retinal fluid. Specifically, employing microperimetry in acute CSCR eyes aided in the identification of persistent sub-retinal fluid allowing earlier intervention to possibly prevent long-term damage [51]. Microperimetry in combination with scanning laser ophthalmoscopy [52] can be considered for the detection and management of CSCR in addition to the prevention of a chronic disease state resulting from CSCR.

EFFECTS OF THERAPY ON THE DIAGNOSIS OF CSCR

CSCR is often clinically manifested as a serous retinal detachment associated with increased blood vessel permeability throughout the choriocapillaris. Current standard of care therapy for CSCR involves treatment with corticosteroids, spironolactone, and acetazolamide, as well as photodynamic therapy and intravitreal anti-vascular endothelial growth factor (VEGF) therapy. Corticosteroid treatment for CSCR is reported to have varying effects. In the study by Prakash and colleagues, a patient, who receiving topical dexamethasone showed complete resolution [53]. Corticosteroid therapy, however, has also been observed to aggravate CSCR disease phenotypes. Corticosteroid administration often leads to termination of its use as an essential initial approach in the treatment [54]. Treatment of CSCR with spironolactone based diuretics, such as eplerenone, decreases sub-foveal fluid volume as well as choroidal thickness resulting in an improvement in visual function in CSCR patients [55]. Such mineralocorticoid receptor antagonism is often pursued as a CSCR therapeutic approach to resolve structural and functional deficiencies in CSCR as CSCR could be caused by abnormally overactive mineralocorticoid receptor pathways in the retinal blood vessels [56]. Pharmacotherapy of CSCR patients with acetazolamide have also resulted in a partial decrease in choroidal thickness to normal reference parameters [57].

Half-dose photodynamic therapy has been a successful treatment option for CSCR leading to improved visual acuity and contrast sensitivity and a decrease in central foveal thickness [58]. Similarly, reduced-fluence photodynamic therapy generates a decrease in macular choroidal thickness within six months of treatment [59] while photodynamic therapy results in complete resolution of sub-retinal fluid build-up and PED [60]. In this context, assessments of mean choroidal thickness, and diameter of diseased choroidal blood vessels, are useful tools to determine the efficacy of photodynamic therapy in CSCR [61]. Photodynamic therapy can be monitored effectively with diagnostic methods and can be adjusted to achieve the best possible treatment outcome while minimizing side effects [62]. The use of low dose verteporfin may compliment safe and effective photodynamic therapy for CSCR and produce long-term resolution of CSCR symptoms without generating retinal atrophy [63]. Photodynamic therapy, when combined with intravitreally delivered anti-VEGF therapy, can produce optimized treatment options for CSCR and result in the resolution of macular neurosensory retinal detachment, improved vision and decreased reoccurrence [64].

Intravitreal aflibercept injections have been reported to reduce abnormally enlarged central macular thickness as well as the volume of sub-foveal fluid within a period of six months, but did not necessarily improve visual acuity [65]. Anti-VEGF therapy, with intravitreal injections of bevacizumab, improved CSCR only in a subset of patients with less severe disease [66]. Another study on patients with anti-VEGF therapy found broader improvements in choroidal thickness and blood flood flow, as well as a reduction in sub-retinal fluid volume [67]. Semeraro and colleagues found that intravitreal injections of bevacizumab represent a superior treatment for CSCR than photodynamic therapy based on an improvement in visual acuity [68]. While the determination of long-term effects of intravitreal anti-VEGF therapy as a treatment for CSCR may require more studies, it represents a valuable treatment modality for the care of CSCR patients [69].

Clinical Trials

With an increase in CSCR prevalence, there is a growing need for research and clinical trials. The completed clinical trial, Comparison of Multifocal Electroretinogram Assessment in Chronic Central Serous Chorioretinopathy (CSC) Between Laser Treatment Group and Photodynamic Therapy Group in Chronic Central Serous Chorioretinopathy [70], used multifocal ERGs to determine that focal laser photocoagulation was superior to photodynamic therapy in restoring ERG amplitudes and in improving visual acuity in CSCR. A one-year study comparing intravitreal ranibizumab to low-fluence photodynamic therapy [71] concluded that more patients had complete resolution of sub-retinal fluid buildup in the low-fluence photodynamic therapy group. In addition to these recently completed clinical trials, [72] is evaluating the reproducibility of microperimetry as part of Spectral OCT/SLO assessments in the diagnosis of CSCR. While microperimetry is generally a reliable diagnostic tool for detecting CSCR, additional research is needed as microperimetry since it identifies abnormal retinal function in individuals without retinal disease. The completed clinical trial, Extension Study for the

Evaluation of Finasteride in the Treatment of Chronic CSCR, identified finasteride as an effective short-term treatment for CSCR without improvement of visual acuity long-term [73]. These completed clinical trials, as well as a range of other clinical trials, on CSCR treatment and diagnostics [74-78] generally prompt the need for improved diagnostics technology and protocols.

SUMMARY/OUTLOOK

CSCR diagnosis remains difficult in the absence of sufficiently accurate and specific diagnostic technology and, while current diagnostic methods seem to facilitate differential diagnosis of CSCR, better strategies are needed to diagnose the acute stages of the disease in order to distinguish between inflammatory and non-inflammatory conditions of the retina. Current diagnostic methods are able to detect leakage and buildup of sub-retinal fluid and retinal atrophy resulting from the hyper-permeability of choroid blood vessels, additional parameters are needed, however, in order to more accurately distinguish CSCR from other conditions [1-4]. Other factors such as altered choroid vascularization and the absence of inflammatory factors could also be used as novel diagnostic targets. While the treatment of CSCR has continued to improve and includes selective retinal therapies, which can precisely target RPE cells and RPE leaks without adversely affecting the neural retina, additional therapies need development requiring also improved diagnostic methods [1-4]. Such new treatment approaches currently under development and in clinical trials range from identifying the role of pathogens in CSCR disease development to evaluating the therapeutic value of antioxidants and intravitreal anti-VEGF therapies and outcomes of such trials are invariably tied to high-quality diagnostics.

REFERENCES

[1] Wang, M, Munch, IC, Hasler PW, et al. Central Serous Chorioretinopathy. *Acta Ophthalmol* (2008) 86. 2, 126-45.

[2] Gemenetzi, M., G. De Salvo, and A. J. Lotery. "Central Serous Chorioretinopathy: An Update on Pathogenesis and Treatment." *Eye* 24.12 (2010): 1743-756.

[3] Marina Papadia MD, PhD, Bruno Jeannin CRO, Carl P Herbort MD, PhD. Central serous chorioretinopathy misdiagnosed as posterior uveitis and the vicious circle of corticosteroid therapy. *Journal of Ophthalmic & Vision Research*. 26 November 2015 Volume 10, page 303-308.

[4] Kang, Seungbum MD, PhD; Park, Young Gun MD; Kim, Jae Ryun MD; Seifert, Eric MS; Theisen-Kunde, Dirk MS; Brinkmann, Ralf PhD; Roh, Young Jung MD, PhD. *Selective Retina Therapy in Patients With Chronic Central Serous Chorioretinopathy: A Pilot Study*. Medicine. January 2016 Volume 95, page 1-9.

[5] Yang, L., Jonas, J. B. and Wei, W. Choroidal vessel diameter in central serous chorioretinopathy. *Acta Ophthalmologica*. 7 May 2013 Volume 91, pages e358-e362.

[6] George J. Manayath, Saurabh Arora, Hardik Parikh, Parag K. Shah, Sarvesh Tiwari, and Venkatapathy Narendran. Is myopia a protective factor against central serous chorioretinopathy?. *International Journal of Ophthalmology*. 18 February 2016 Volume 9, page 266-270.

[7] Woo Beom Shin, Min Kyo Kim, Christopher Seungkyu Lee, Sung Chul Lee, and Hyesun Kim. Comparison of the Clinical Manifestations between Acute Vogt-Koyanagi-Harada Disease and Acute Bilateral Central Serous Chorioretinopathy. *Korean Journal of Ophthalmology*. 25 November 2015 Volume 29, page 389-395.

[8] Sang Hoon Jung PhD, Kyung-A Kim MS, Sea Woon Sohn MD, and Sung Jae Yang MD. Cytokine levels of the aqueous humour in central serous chorioretinopathy. *Clinical and Experimental Optometry*. 14 January 2014 Volume 97, page 264-269.

[9] Marcuson, J., and Riley T. "Central Serous Chorioretinopathy." *Optometry* 79.5 (2008): 241-51.

[10] Conway, Mandi D., Jason A. Noble, and Gholam A. Peyman. "Central Serous Chorioretinopathy In Postmenopausal Women Receiving Exogenous Testosterone." Retinal Cases & Brief Reports (2016): 1.

[11] Perkins, Stephen L., Judy E. Kim, John S. Pollack, and Pauline T. Merrill. "Clinical Characteristics of Central Serous Chorioretinopathy in Women." *Ophthalmology* 109.2 (2002): 262-66.

[12] Weenink, AC., RA. Borsje, and JA. Oosterhuis. "Familial Chronic Central Serous Chorioretinopathy." *Ophthalmologica* 215.3 (2001): 183-87.

[13] Desai, UR., AA. Alhalel, TJ. Campen, RM. Schiffman, PA. Edwards, and GR. Jacobsen. "Central Serous Chorioretinopathy in African Americans." *J Natl Med Assoc*. 95.7 (2003): 553-59.

[14] Pare, Joseph R., Yan Guo, and Elissa M. Schechter-Perkins. "The Evaluation of Acute Vision Loss: Central Serous Chorioretinopathy." *The American Journal of Emergency Medicine* 32.4 (2014).

[15] Fujita, K., K. Shinoda, CS. Matsumoto, Y. Imamura, Y. Mizutani, E. Tanaka, A. Mizota, K. Oda, and M. Yuzawa. "Low Luminance Visual Acuity in Patients with Central Serous Chorioretiinopathy." *Clin. Exp. Optom.* 96.1 (2013): 100-05.

[16] Wang, MS., B. Sander, and M. Larsen. "Retinal Atrophy in Idiopathic Central Serous Chorioretinopathy." *Eye (Lond) 27*.5 (2013): 612-20.

[17] Lee, K., J. Sohn, J. G. Choi, and S. K. Chung. "Optical Quality in Central Serous Chorioretinopathy." *Investigative Ophthalmology & Visual Science* 55.12 (2014): 8598-603.

[18] Plainis, S., AG. Anastasakis, and MK. Tsilimbaris. "The Value of Contrast Sensitivity in Diagnosing Central Serous Chorioretinopathy." *Int. Ophthalmol.* 23.1 (1999): 31-35.

[19] Bartos, D., J. Kondrova, V. Stibor, L. Bartosova, and A. Rousova. "Changes in Psychovisual Function after Central Serous Chorioretinopathy." *Surv. Ophthalmol.* 58.2 (2013): 103-26.

[20] Nicholson, Benjamin, Jason Noble, Farzin Forooghian, and Catherine Meyerle. "Central Serous Chorioretinopathy: Update on Pathophysiology and Treatment." *Survey of Ophthalmology* 58.2 (2013): 103-26.

[21] Hua, Rui, Kai Yao, Fan Xia, Jun Li, Lei Guo, Guoxing Yang, and Jun Tao. "The Hyper-fluorescent Transitional Bands in Ultra-late Phase of Indocyanine Green Angiography in Chronic Central Serous Chorioretinopathy." *Lasers Surg. Med. Lasers in Surgery and Medicine* 48.3 (2015): 260-63.

[22] Gajdzik-Gajdecka, Urszula, Mariola Dorecka, Ewa Nita, Anna Michalska, Joanna Miniewicz-Kurowska, and Wanda Romaniuk. "Indocyanine Green Angiography in Chronic Central Serous Chorioretinopathy." *Med Sci Monit Medical Science Monitor* 18.2 (2012): n. pag.

[23] Tsujikawa, Akitaka, Yumiko Ojima, Kenji Yamashiro, Sotaro Ooto, Hiroshi Tamura, Satoko Nakagawa, and Nagahisa Yoshimura. "Punctate Hyperfluorescent Spots Associated With Central Serous Chorioretinopathy As Seen On Indocyanine Green Angiography." *Retina* 30.5 (2010): 801-09.

[24] Pang, Claudine E., Vinnie P. Shah, David Sarraf, and K. Bailey Freund. "Ultra-Widefield Imaging With Autofluorescence and Indocyanine

Green Angiography in Central Serous Chorioretinopathy." *American Journal of Ophthalmology* 158.2 (2014): n. pag.

[25] Ricci, F., F. Missiroli, F. Regine, M. Grossi, and G. Dorin. "Indocyanine Green Enhanced Subthreshold Diode-laser Micropulse Photocoagulation Treatment of Chronic Central Serous Chorioretinopathy." *Graefes Arch Clin Exp Ophthalmol Graefe's Archive for Clinical and Experimental Ophthalmology* 247.5 (2008): 597-607.

[26] Teussink, Michel M., Myrte B. Breukink, Mark J. J. P. Van Grinsven, Carel B. Hoyng, B. Jeroen Klevering, Camiel J. F. Boon, Eiko K. De Jong, and Thomas Theelen. "OCT Angiography Compared to Fluorescein and Indocyanine Green Angiography in Chronic Central Serous Chorioretinopathy." *Invest. Ophthalmol.* Vis. Sci. 56.9 (2015): 5229.

[27] Mrejen, Sarah, and Richard F. Spaide. "Optical Coherence Tomography: Imaging of the Choroid and beyond." *Survey of Ophthalmology* 58.5 (2013): 387-429.

[28] Hee MR, Puliafito CA, Wong C, Reichel E, Duker JS, Schuman JS, Swanson EA, Fujimoto JG.. "Optical Coherence Tomography of Central Serous Chorioretinopathy." *American Journal Ophthalmology* 120.1 (1995): 65-74.

[29] Maftouhi, Maddalena Quaranta-El, Adil El Maftouhi, and Chiara M. Eandi. "Chronic Central Serous Chorioretinopathy Imaged by Optical Coherence Tomographic Angiography." *American Journal of Ophthalmology* 160.3 (2015): n. pag.

[30] Iida, T., N. Hagimura, T. Sato, and S. Kishi. "Evaluation of Central Serous Chorioretinopathy with Optical Coherence Tomography." *American Journal of Ophthalmology* 129.1 (2000): 16-20.

[31] Sander, B., M. Larsen, L. Thrane, JL. Hougaard, and TM. Jørgensen. "Enhanced Optical Coherence Tomography Imaging by Multiple Scan Averaging." *British Journal of Ophthalmology* 89.2 (2005): 207-12.

[32] Carrai, Paola, Francesco Pichi, Francesco Bonsignore, Antonio P. Ciardella, and Paolo Nucci. "Wide-field Spectral Domain-optical Coherence Tomography in Central Serous Chorioretinopathy." *International Ophthalmology Int Ophthalmol* 35.2 (2015): 167-71

[33] Salvo, Gabriella De, Sara Vaz-Pereira, Pearse A. Keane, Adnan Tufail, and Gerald Liew. "Sensitivity and Specificity of Spectral-Domain Optical Coherence Tomography in Detecting Idiopathic Polypoidal Choroidal Vasculopathy." *American Journal of Ophthalmology* 158.6 (2014): n. pag.

[34] Hata, Masayuki, Akio Oishi, Masataka Shimozono, Michiko Mandai, Akihiro Nishida, and Yasuo Kurimoto. "Early Changes in Foveal Thickness In Eyes With Central Serous Chorioretinopathy." *Retina* 33.2 (2013): 296-301.

[35] Furuta, Minoru, Tomohiro Iida, and Shoji Kishi. "Foveal Thickness Can Predict Visual Outcome in Patients with Persistent Central Serous Chorioretinopathy." *Ophthalmologica* 223.1 (2009): 28-31.

[36] Aggio, Fabio B., Luiz Roisman, Gustavo B. Melo, Daniel Lavinsky, José A. Cardillo, and Michel E. Farah. "Clinical Factors Related To Visual Outcome In Central Serous Chorioretinopathy." *Retina* 30.7 (2010): 1128-134.

[37] Byon, Ik Soo, Hyun Jun Park, Sung Who Park, Kyung Ho Kim, Ji Eun Lee, and Boo Sub Oum. "Tissue Layer Image of the Photoreceptor Layer in Central Serous Chorioretinopathy Using SD-OCT." *Ophthalmic Surg Lasers Imaging Ophthalmic Surgery, Lasers, and Imaging* 43.6 (2012): n. pag.

[38] Flores, Mathieu, Guillaume Debellemanière, Alois Bully, Mathieu Meillat, Perle Tumahai, Bernard Delbosc, and Maher Saleh. "Reflectivity of the Outer Retina on Spectral-Domain Optical Coherence Tomography As a Predictor of Photoreceptor Cone Density." *American Journal of Ophthalmology* 160.3 (2015): n. pag.

[39] Saito, M., W. Saito, Y. Hashimoto, C. Yoshizawa, A. Fujiya, K. Noda, and S. Ishida. "Macular Choroidal Blood Flow Velocity Decreases with Regression of Acute Central Serous Chorioretinopathy." *British Journal of Ophthalmology* 97.6 (2013): 775-80.

[40] Saito, Michiyuki, Wataru Saito, Kiriko Hirooka, Yuki Hashimoto, Shohei Mori, Kousuke Noda, and Susumu Ishida. "Pulse Waveform Changes in Macular Choroidal Hemodynamics With Regression of Acute Central Serous Chorioretinopathy." Investigative Opthalmology & Visual Science Invest. *Ophthalmol. Vis. Sci.* 56.11 (2015): 6515.

[41] Sugiyama, Tetsuya, Makoto Araie, Charles E. Riva, Leopold Schmetterer, and Selim Orgul. "Use of Laser Speckle Flowgraphy in Ocular Blood Flow Research." *Acta Ophthalmologica* 88.7 (2009): 723-29.

[42] Kitaya, N. "Features of Abnormal Choroidal Circulation in Central Serous Chorioretinopathy." *British Journal of Ophthalmology* 87.6 (2003): 709-12.

[43] Suzuki, K. "Multifocal Electroretinogram in Patients with Central Serous Chorioretinopathy." *Japanese Journal of Ophthalmology* 46.3 (2002): 308-14.

[44] Goyal, Jawahar Lal, Basudeb Ghosh, Vishram Sangit, Sushil Kumar, Parul Jain, Vikas Veerwal, and Ritu Arora. "Pattern ERG in Central Serous Retinopathy." *Documenta Ophthalmologica* 130.2 (2014): 141-47.

[45] Moschos, Marilita, Dimitrios Brouzas, Chrysanthi Koutsandrea, Baltatzis Stefanos, Heleni Loukianou, Fotis Papantonis, and Michael Moschos. "Assessment of Central Serous Chorioretinopathy by Optical Coherence Tomography and Multifocal Electroretinography." *Ophthalmologica* 221.5 (2007): 292-98.

[46] Ozdemir, H., F. Senturk, M. Karacorlu, S. Arf Karacorlu, and O. Uvsal. "Macular Sensitivity in Eyes with Central Serous Chorioretinopathy." *Eur. J. Ophthalmol* 18.5 (2008): 799-804.

[47] Eandi, Chiara M., Felice Cardillo Piccolino, Camilla Alovisi, Federico Tridico, Daniela Giacomello, and Federico M. Grignolo. "Correlation Between Fundus Autofluorescence and Central Visual Function in Chronic Central Serous Chorioretinopathy." *Am J Ophthalmol.* 2015 Apr;159(4):652-8.

[48] Chung, H. W., C. M. Yun, J. T. Kim, S-W Kim, J. Oh, and K. Huh. "Retinal Sensitivity Assessed by Microperimetry and Corresponding Retinal Structure and Thickness in Resolved Central Serous Chorioretinopathy." *Eye* 28.10 (2014): 1223-1230.

[49] Schliesser JA, Gallimore G, Kunjukunju N, Sabates NR, Koulen P, Sabates FN. Clinical application of optical coherence tomography in combination with functional diagnostics: advantages and limitations for diagnosis and assessment of therapy outcome in central serous chorioretinopathy. *Clin Ophthalmol.* 2014 Nov 21;8:2337-45.

[50] Sabates FN, Vincent RD, Koulen P, Sabates NR, Gallimore G. Normative data set identifying properties of the macula across age groups: integration of visual function and retinal structure with microperimetry and spectral-domain optical coherence tomography. *Retina.* 2011 Jul-Aug;31(7):1294-302.

[51] Roisman, Luiz, João C. Ribeiro, Francisco V. Fechine, Daniel Lavinsky, Nilva Moraes, Mauro Campos, and Michel E. Farah. "Does Microperimetry Have A Prognostic Value In Central Serous Chorioretinopathy?" *Retina* 34.4 (2014): 713-18.

[52] Rohrschneider, Klaus, Christina Springer, Stefan Bültmann, and Hans E. Völcker. "Microperimetry — Comparison between the Micro Perimeter 1 and Scanning Laser Ophthalmoscope — Fundus Perimetry." *American Journal of Ophthalmology* 139.1 (2005): 125-34.

[53] Prakash, Gunjan, Jain Shephali, Nath Tirupati, and Pandeyd Ji. "Recurrent Central Serous Chorioretinopathy with Dexamethasone Eye Drop Used Nasally for Rhinitis." *Middle East African Journal of Ophthalmology Middle East Afr J Ophthalmol* 20.4 (2013): 363.

[54] Khairallah, M., R. Kahloun, and I. Tugal-tutkun. "Central Serous Chorioretinopathy, Corticosteroids, and Uveitis." *Ocul. Immunol Inflamm.* 20.2 (2012): 76-85.

[55] Salz, David A., John D. Pitcher, Jason Hsu, Carl D. Regillo, Mitchell S. Fineman, Kevin S. Elliott, James F. Vander, David H. Fischer, and Marc J. Spirn. "Oral Eplerenone for Treatment of Chronic Central Serous Chorioretinopathy: A Case Series." *Ophthalmic Surgery, Lasers and Imaging Retina Ophthalmic Surg Lasers Imaging Retina* 46.4 (2015): 439-44.

[56] Bousquet, Elodie, Talal Beydoun, Min Zhao, Leila Hassan, Olivier Offret, and Francine Behar-Cohen. "Mineralocorticoid Receptor Antagonism In The Treatment Of Chronic Central Serous Chorioretinopathy." *Retina* 33.10 (2013): 2096-102.

[57] Brandl, Caroline, H. Helbig, and M. A. Gamulescu. "Choroidal Thickness Measurements during Central Serous Chorioretinopathy Treatment." *International Ophthalmology Int Ophthalmol* 34.1 (2013): 7-13.

[58] Karakus, S. H., B. Basarir, E. Y. Pinarci, E. U. Kirandi, and A. Demirok. "Long-term Results of Half-dose Photodynamic Therapy for Chronic Central Serous Chorioretinopathy with Contrast Sensitivity Changes." *Eye* 27.5 (2013): 612-20.

[59] Manabe, Saki, Chieko Shiragami, Kazuyuki Hirooka, Saeko Izumibata, Akitaka Tsujikawa, and Fumio Shiraga. "Change of Regional Choroid Thickness After Reduced-Fluence Photodynamic Therapy for Chronic Central Serous Chorioretinopathy." *American Journal of Ophthalmology* 159.4 (2015): n. pag.

[60] Tsai, Meng-Ju, and Yi-Ting Hsieh. "Half-Time Photodynamic Therapy for Central Serous Chorioretinopathy." *Optometry and Vision Science* 91.9 (2014): 1140-145.

[61] Hua, Rui, Limin Liu, Chenyan Li, and Lei Chen. "Evaluation of the Effects of Photodynamic Therapy on Chronic Central Serous

Chorioretinopathy Based on the Mean Choroidal Thickness and the Lumen Area of Abnormal Choroidal Vessels." *Photodiagnosis and Photodynamic Therapy* 11.4 (2014): 519-25.

[62] Ma, Jinlan, Nana Meng, Xiaoyi Xu, Fang Zhou, and Yi Qu. "System Review and Meta-analysis on Photodynamic Therapy in Central Serous Chorioretinopathy." *Acta Ophthalmologica Acta Ophthalmol* 92.8 (2014): n. pag.

[63] Zhao, Ming-Wei, Peng Zhou, Hong-Xiang Xiao, Yong-Shun Lv, Chun-An Li, Guo-Dong Liu, and Xiao-Xin Li. " Photodynamic therapy for acute central serous chorioretinopathy: the safe effective lowest dose of verteporfin." *Retina* 29.8 (2009): 1155-161.

[64] Arevalo, J. Fernando, and Juan V. Espinoza. "Single-session Combined Photodynamic Therapy with Verteporfin and Intravitreal Anti-vascular Endothelial Growth Factor Therapy for Chronic Central Serous Chorioretinopathy: A Pilot Study at 12-month Follow-up." *Graefes Arch Clin Exp Ophthalmol Graefe's Archive for Clinical and Experimental Ophthalmology* 249.8 (2011): 1159-166.

[65] Pitcher, John D., Andre J. Witkin, Francis Char Decroos, and Allen C. Ho. "A Prospective Pilot Study of Intravitreal Aflibercept for the Treatment of Chronic Central Serous Chorioretinopathy: The CONTAIN Study." *British Journal of Ophthalmology Br J Ophthalmol* 99.6 (2015): 848-52.

[66] Kim, G. A., T. H. Rim, S. C. Lee, S. H. Byeon, H. J. Koh, S. S. Kim, and C. S. Lee. "Clinical Characteristics of Responders to Intravitreal Bevacizumab in Central Serous Chorioretinopathy Patients." *Eye* 29.6 (2015): 732-41.

[67] Okamoto, Masahiro, Toyoaki Matsuura, and Nahoko Ogata. "Choroidal Thickness and Choroidal Blood Flow after Intravitreal Bevacizumab Injection in Eyes with Central Serous Chorioretinopathy." *Ophthalmic Surgery, Lasers and Imaging Retina Ophthalmic Surg Lasers Imaging Retina* 46.1 (2015): 25-32.

[68] Semeraro, Francesco, Mario R. Romano, Paola Danzi, Francesco Morescalchi, and Ciro Costagliola. "Intravitreal Bevacizumab versus Low-fluence Photodynamic Therapy for Treatment of Chronic Central Serous Chorioretinopathy." *Japanese Journal of Ophthalmology Jpn J Ophthalmol* 56.6 (2012): 608-12.

[69] Lee, Shelly T., and Ron A. Adelman. "The Treatment of Recurrent Central Serous Chorioretinopathy with Intravitreal Bevacizumab." *Journal of Ocular Pharmacology and Therapeutics* 27.6 (2011): 611-14.

[70] https://clinicaltrials.gov/ct2/show/NCT00803517?term=Central+Serous+Chorioretinopathy&rank=9.
[71] https://clinicaltrials.gov/ct2/show/NCT01325181?term=Central+Serous+Chorioretinopathy&rank=20.
[72] https://clinicaltrials.gov/ct2/show/NCT01692938?term=Central+Serous+Chorioretinopathy&rank=49.
[73] https://clinicaltrials.gov/ct2/show/NCT01227993?term=Central+Serous+Chorioretinopathy&rank=28.
[74] https://clinicaltrials.gov/ct2/show/NCT01378130?term=Central+Serous+Chorioretinopathy%3A+Etiology%2C+Course+and+Prognosis&rank=1.
[75] https://clinicaltrials.gov/ct2/show/NCT01019668?term=Central+Serous+Chorioretinopathy&rank=6.
[76] https://clinicaltrials.gov/ct2/show/NCT01327170?term=Central+Serous+Chorioretinopathy&rank=11.
[77] https://clinicaltrials.gov/ct2/show/NCT01971190?term=Central+Serous+Chorioretinopathy&rank=23.
[78] https://clinicaltrials.gov/ct2/show/NCT00802906?term=Central+Serous+Chorioretinopathy&rank=34.

BIOGRAPHICAL SKETCH

Name: Peter Koulen

Affiliation: Vision Research Center, Department of Ophthalmology and Department of Basic Medical Science, University of Missouri – Kansas City, School of Medicine

Education: PhD

Address: University of Missouri – Kansas City, School of Medicine, 2411 Holmes St., Kansas City, MO 64108, US

Research and Professional Experience: Co-Director and Director of Basic Research, Vision Research Center, University of Missouri - Kansas City, School of Medicine

Professional Appointments: Professor of Ophthalmology, Cell Biology and Biophysics, and Basic Medical Sciences

Honors: Felix and Carmen Sabates Missouri Endowed Chair in Vision Research

Publications: http://www.ncbi.nlm.nih.gov/sites/myncbi/peter.koulen.1/bibliography/45925425/public/?sort=date&direction=descending.

In: Central Serous Chorioretinopathy (CSCR) ISBN: 978-1-53610-806-4
Editor: Patrick Evans

Chapter 3

SUBTHRESHOLD MICROPULSE LASER THERAPY IN CENTRAL SEROUS CHORIORETINOPATHY

Federico Ortiz-Coto[1,*], MD, Alonso Gutierrez-Guerinoni[2], MD and Juan Carlos Gutierrez-Hernandez[3], MD

[1]Clinica Oftalmocima; Caja Costarricense del Seguro Social, San Jose, Costa Rica

[2]Department of Ophthalmology, Universidad de Costa Rica, San Jose, Costa Rica

[3]Hospital Clinica Biblica; Caja Costarricense del Seguro Social, San Jose, Costa Rica

ABSTRACT

The pathogenesis of central serous choroidopathy (CSCR) is a complex one, in which there is a choroidal dysfunction that leads a hyperpermeability state of the choroid and a retinal pigment epithelium (RPE) detachment and leakage of fluid into the sub retinal space, affecting the posterior pole. It has been associated with high levels of corticosteroids, both endogenous and exogenous, Helicobacter pylori

[*] Corresponding author: fortizcmd@gmail.com.

infections, Type-A personalities, but in the majority it has an idiopathic origin.

Two subtypes have been described, acute CSCR and chronic CSCR. It has a usually benign natural history; it resolves without treatment usually within four to six months. In the acute phases, usually a focal leakage point can be seen on both the fluorescein angiography (FA) and indocyanine-green angiography (IGA). In chronic or recurrent cases, usually there is no focal, but a diffuse area of leakage that spreads over a wider area of the posterior pole. Extra foveal focal leakage points can be and have been treated in the past with conventional laser photocoagulation to expedite the resolution of the serous detachment, but the final visual acuity (VA) is often the same as that with spontaneous healing. The way laser works is not fully understood, although it is aimed in destroying and scarring leaking vessels with a theoretical healthy RPE cell migration that takes over the pump function. Several complications have been identified with this treatment, which include scotomas, choroidal neovascularization (CNV), retinal scarring, and contrast sensitivity. Because of these reasons, this treatment is considered ideally for patients with recurrent or chronic cases, those with permanent CSCR changes in the fellow eye, or a professional need for a quick recovery by the patient. Other treatments include anti vascular endothelial growth factor agents (anti-VEGF) as well as photodynamic therapy (PDT). PDT is not exempt from developing many of the complications as conventional laser therapy, thus leading to the development of new technologies for the treatment of macular diseases, amongst which subthreshold micropulse laser therapy of the RPE has shown results comparable to those of conventional laser therapy.

Preliminary studies with the micropulse technology were with 810nm laser, although 577nm yellow laser has stood out in recent practices. In micropulse mode, laser is delivered in short pulses that allow for a cooling of the tissues in between these. Conventional laser causes a photocoagulative effect on the neurosensory retina with a surrounding area of treatment around each burn. Micropulse laser on the other hand, creates a photothermal effect that stimulates the RPE the retinal without the burn or scarring of the neurosensory retina. This reaction is only distinguished in histological and microscopical examination, but is otherwise undetectable. Yellow laser is poorly absorbed by the xanthophyll pigment mostly found on the fovea, which allows a transfoveal treatment. Few adverse effects have been reported with the use of this laser, being retinal edema and SRF the most commonly reported. Subthreshold micropulse laser therapy presents as a treatment option for those cases in which the fovea is involved.

Keywords: central serous chorioretinopathy, subthreshold micropulse laser, treatment

INTRODUCTION

Central serous chorioretinopathy has been first described in the 19th century by Albert von Graefe and since has been given various nomenclatures [1] [2]. Currently, the term most commonly used is Central Serous Chorioretinopathy, a term Gass JD used to describe a disciform detachment of the neurosensory retina in 1967 [3]. It is characterized by a neurosensory retinal detachment of the retina. CSCR is the fourth most common retinopathy behind age related macular degeneration, diabetic retinopathy, and retinal vein occlusions [4]. Since then, several treatments have been used to treat this pathology with mixed results. There are no treatment guidelines approved for this disease as it usually is self-limited with a good visual recovery over three to six months. Despite this, between one third to half of the cases have some degree of visual impairment, especially in chronic cases [5] [6] [7]. New treatment options are currently being developed for these patients, as well as those with permanent visual loss due to CSCR in the fellow eye, or those patients with an urgent need for visual recovery. Both acute and chronic CSCR have been described. Chronic CSCR has been defined by some authors as three months, while others define it as six months. In this group of patients, laser therapy has been used to accelerate the rate of recovery of these patients since the late seventies and well into the eighties, although there has been no strong evidence to support any changes in the final visual outcome [8] [9]. Usually in these cases there can be seen, both on FA and ICG, a focal leakage point, into which the treatment is guided to. Autofluorescence also shows both leakage areas as well as the areas of sub retinal fluid as both hyperautofluorescent and hypoautofluorescent areas on the retina, respectively [10]. Optical coherence tomography (OCT), also shows the characteristic neurosensory retinal detachment with the sub retinal fluid. New angiography OCT demonstrated a high intensity signal with dilated choriocapillaris vessels in patients diagnosed with CSCR [11].

LASER THERAPY IN CSCR

Lasers have diverse applications in the treatment of retinal and macular diseases, amongst which CSCR is found. Laser treatment relies on the characteristics of monochromatism, coherence, and directionality [12]. A photon stimulates an excited atom to stimulate a release of a second photon, which is uniform in frequency and phase as the first photon (stimulated emission). This creates a chain reaction of stimulated emission in which the excitation phase is greater than the rate of decay of atoms into a lower energy state. This energy is enclosed in the laser system by mirrors, which also gives them directionality into a single direction. Both argon and krypton laser have been tested throughout the years with different laser patterns used, such as direct photocoagulation of the leakage site, as well as grid photocoagulation [8] [9] [13] [14]. Visual side effects have been described for different types of laser treatment, which include moderate visual field loss, diminished contrast sensitivity, reduced color vision, formation of sub retinal choroidal neovascular membranes, and both retinal and foveal scarring [15] [16]. Subthreshold micropulse laser therapy technology, introduced in the last decade, has come to address the possible complications of conventional laser treatments based on the effect of the specific yellow wavelength on the macular pigments and tissues. Several wavelengths have been tested, with 577nm yellow laser being the predominant wavelength utilized in recent years.

Current practices dictate observation as the first line of treatment. Treatment using laser photocoagulation may be indicated in the following cases [17]:

- Persistent CSCR beyond 3-6 months.
- Recurring disease in eyes with visual deficit from previous episodes.
- Permanent visual defect in fellow eye from a previous episode.
- Chronic changes in neurosensory retina and/or RPE.
- Occupational or personal visual needs which require prompt resolution.

PREVIOUS LASER AND CSCR

Xenon Arc

Xenon arc technology consists of a high pressure light bulb that delivers energy from all the wavelengths in the visible light spectrum, as well as near infrared wavelengths. This very broad light spectrum is absorbed by almost all the ocular tissues, and can have a photocoagulative effect on them. Xenon arc delivers high energy levels to all the tissues, while conventional laser therapy targets only the pigmented tissues [18]. Initial studies for diabetic retinopathy showed similar results in visual acuity and efficacy as argon laser, although it produced more adverse effects in comparison, especially visual field loss and night vision [18] [19] [20]. Furthermore, it was difficult to focus the laser beam into a small spot, required a long time, and in occasions was painful for patients.

Ruby Laser

One of the first lasers utilized to treat CSCR was the ruby laser, with a 694nm laser wavelength emission [21] [22]. Watzke et al. in 1974 reported a series of cases treated with ruby laser, which had remission and improvement of both subretinal fluid, and improvement in visual acuity within five weeks after treatment. Ruby laser emits a light near the red spectrum of light wavelength, and theoretically has a greater absorption in the choroid and choriocapillaris layers, with little to no absorption by hemoglobin in the blood vessels [23]. This would prevent any damage on other structures, and would target one of the proposed specific area of pathology in CSCR. Being one of the first lasers, it has now been surpassed by modern laser systems due to severe damage to the choroid and frequent hemorrhaging.

Krypton Laser

Krypton laser consists of a red laser with a wavelength of 810nm with tissue selectivity for the retinal pigment epithelium. For this reason, it was first considered in the treatment of CSCR [13]. Furthermore, the macular pigment and the capillary beds of the inner retinal layers have an inability to absorb this wavelength, further supporting krypton laser as a treatment option [13]. Patients treated tended to have a more rapid recovery and fewer recurrences, even when compared with argon laser treatment initially [13] [24] [25]. Several complications have been reported associated with krypton laser, with a significant visual loss rate of over three percent of cases treated. Most reports with complications are when it is utilized as treatment for other macular diseases such as subretinal neovascular membranes, and diabetic maculopathy

[26]. Significant choroidal hemorrhages, along with RPE breaks are the most common visually significant complications reported. Other complications such as choroidal ischemia and choroidal folds have also been described [26] [27].

Argon Laser

Argon laser can be green (514nm) or blue (488 nm). The use of argon laser photocoagulation became more prevalent over xenon arc krypton laser due to less frequent visual threatening complications. The Diabetic Retinopathy Study (DRS) demonstrated similar results between argon laser therapy and xenon arc, with fewer complications for argon laser. [20]. Argon laser has proven to hasten the visual recovery of patients, although there is no evidence that it influences the final visual outcome of these [8] [9] [24]. It has also shown to be effective and safe in selected patients. The more serious potential hazards remain to be inadvertent foveal photocoagulation, as well as a strong energy absorption from the macula in these patients [8]. Still, more serious and complicated events have been described such as subretinal choroidal membrane neovascularization, although this has been debated over the years [16]. Other complications reported are scotomas, retinal wrinkling, subretinal hemorrhage and decreased visual acuity [28].

Neodymium Diode and Solid State Lasers

Studies have suggested that the primary site of pathology in this disease is the choroid and choriocapillaris, and not the RPE [29]. Due to this, treatment more focused has been tried to target this specific area. Neodymium-doped yttrium orthovanadate (Nd:YVO_4), as well as a double sequenced neodymium-doped yttrium lithium fluoride (Nd:YLF) and yttrium aluminum garnet (Nd: YAG) laser have been tested for treatment of various retinal diseases. These use neodymium as a solid-state crystalline medium for diode lasers. It delivers a green laser in a doubled frequency 527nm and 532nm low intensity matter, either in a single pulse mode, or in a series of uniform pulses [30] [31] [32]. Studies involving the use of 532nm green wavelength for various diseases have reported favorable results. Similar to argon laser photocoagulation, it has shown a decrease in the recovery time of patients, without affecting the final visual outcome. Few complications are reported, metamorphopsias being the most common symptom [33]. Histopathological findings have shown a separation of the neurosensory retina from the RPE, as well as severe disruption of the retinal structures and damage to the RPE in animal models [30]. Larger wavelengths penetrate more, therefore diode laser 810nm has been used to treat these cases, and was first studied before more recent wavelengths, such as 532nm and 577nm. In recent times, 577nm yellow laser has gained popularity because it allows a better titration of power in comparison with the 810nm and 532nm. In comparison with argon laser, with diode laser treatment, it has been reported a more rapid visual recovery after treatment [34]. Furthermore, diode laser therapy had less residual scotomas and better contrast sensitivity after treatment. Theoretically, as in targets the primary site of the pathology, it delivers a faster and better qualitative visual recovery from CSCR, while potentially lowering the risk for recurrences and complications, as it is delivered in a low intensity manner [34].

LASER WAVELENGTH

Several factors determine the specific wavelength of light emitted by a laser. These include different media, such as solid state (neodymium:YAG), gases such as argon and krypton, organic dyes, and semiconductors (diode) [35] [36] [37]. The different wavelengths will determine its absorption by the distinct retinal structures and pigments. Therefore, laser wavelength selection must take into consideration the retinal pigments and light absorption characteristics in the desired area in regards with the therapeutic goal for the specific disease. The different pigments have different light wavelength absorption. Melanin, located in the RPE and choroidal melanocytes, has the broadest spectrum of light absorption [38]. The RPE and choroid are aimed at when treating CSCR, therefore it has little influence on wavelength choice [39]. The other pigments have a much narrower light absorption spectrum. Xanthophyll is found in the inner and outer plexiform layers of the retina, and is most present in the macula. It has a poor absorption of yellow laser light, while the hemoglobin present in the retinal blood vessels absorbs it well. Therefore, yellow laser is a good option when treating vascular, RPE and choroidal lesions, while avoiding the uptake on the foveal and macular tissues. Argon blue/green laser is greatly absorbed by xanthophylls, therefore it is not used in focal macular laser treatment, as it will lead to undesired damage to the macular tissues. Red laser light has a decreased absorption compared with the other wavelengths in all pigments and tissues, thus its use as a treatment option is not optimal for posterior segment pathology [38] [40]. The greater the absorption of the laser by the tissue, the greater the thermal effect it will have on the tissue surrounding the laser spot target with retinal scarring.

Micropulse subthreshold laser utilizes a 577nm yellow light wavelength, which targets the specific tissues involved in the CSCR pathophysiology. The RPE, choroid and retinal blood vessels have a good absorption at this light wavelength, sparing the absorption on the macula and retinal tissues. This allows for macular and foveal treatment of lesions. Before, due to the tissue scarring and damage, trans foveal argon laser treatment could not be used in CSCR that involved or threatened the fovea.

Micropulse Principles

Laser has an effect on the different tissues of the retina depending on the power and wavelength utilized [38]. For chorioretinal and vascular pathology, a photocoagulative effect has proven to have beneficial effects on the tissue. It has been suggested that the benefits are due to a regulation of angiogenic growth factor on the retinal pigment epithelium. Conventional laser therapy also produces a destruction of the RPE and photoreceptor cells, diminishing the hypoxia present in the retina. The absorption of conventional argon laser is significant, producing a strong photothermal effect on the different retinal tissues. In conventional photocoagulation, the laser beam is always on throughout the whole duration of the laser shot. The laser energy is absorbed by melanin in the RPE and the choroid. The longer the laser is on, more energy is absorbed in the tissues with heat building up, thus, the photocoagulative effect on the target spot is accompanied by a photothermal effect on the surrounding tissue, leading to excessive scarring with subsequent complications. Conventional laser creates a grayish to white burn on the retina, due to damage of the neurosensory retina. This whitening of the retina is associated with elevated tissue temperatures. Scarring of the retina has association with visual field defects, scotomas, contrast sensitivity, and more severe as retinal fibrosis and formation of neovascular membranes.

The photothermal effect of laser without visible burning of the retina has been studied in the reccnt years, showing a beneficial therapeutic effect [41] [42]. This has been termed subthreshold laser therapy. Subthreshold laser therapy can be obtained modifying the laser parameters to minimize tissue damage. This creates an invisible clinical effect on the retina, with a photothermal stimulation of the RPE. Each micropulse shot consists of a series of repetitive short laser pulses consisting of 100 to 300 microseconds laser

ON, followed by an OFF interval of between 1700-1900 microseconds, enveloped in a 200 to 300 millisecond period of time [43]. Laser power also is markedly reduced to levels even below 50%, still provoking a stimulus to the RPE. The series of short low powered pulses allows a cooling time between them, thus maintaining the temperature below the threshold of photocoagulative damage to the retina. This ensures that no visible damage to the neurosensory retina occurs, and changes can only be found histopathologically or scanning electron microscopy when it is delivered below 50% energy level of a barely visible lesion [44] [45]. A repetitive set of micropulses allows for a lower power utilized in each pulse, with the same beneficial effects on the RPE, thus sparing macular tissue and reducing complications [46]. Subthreshold laser therapy thus can allow retreatment of the macula since there is no permanent damage on the tissues. Nevertheless, concern has risen over the fact that lowering laser energy power in order to minimize collateral tissue damage may result in non-reproducible results on the tissue due to heterogeneity found amongst them on the outer retina and RPE [47].

LASER PARAMETERS

Initial studies proved that when the power is titrated to levels of 50% of the power needed to create a barely visible lesion on the retina, the therapeutic effects are maintained [46]. Laser titration is the most commonly used practice to determine the energy power level to be used. First, power should be increased until a barely visible laser mark on the peripheral normal retina and then, it should be decreased to a 50% power level of that achieved. Kim et al. found that a power level even below 10-20% was enough to produce an effect selectively on the RPE, sparing the neurosensory retina [46]. The most common practice is to deliver laser in a multispot matter with a spot size of 160μm. Zero spacing is used to maximize the treatment area, with an exposure time of 200ms and a duty cycle of 5%. The concept of low intensity, high density is the goal when delivering treatment. Lavinsky et al reported that low intensity, high density patterns in patients with diabetic macular edema (DME) had a larger central macular thickness (CMT) decrease, had a better final best corrected visual acuity, and a larger number of patients with a >15 letter gain [48]. Pattern scan laser treatment has been tested effectively in treatment of CSCR, versus single spot laser therapy, providing a wider area of treatment in a confluent manner [49]. Guided by fluorescein angiography and indocyanine green angiography to identify leakage hotspots, laser is delivered in a multispot confluent pattern. Laser parameter variations can be done, mainly changing the duty cycles and/or spot size, with similar results [50]. Subthreshold laser delivery has a lower diffusion of laser induced heat in the RPE than threshold (visible) laser, producing both less lateral o vertical damage of the retinal structures [51]. Yu et al. demonstrated that subthreshold laser produced no full thickness damage to the retinal structures in comparison with threshold laser at 2 weeks with duty cycles of 40%, 20%, 10% and 5%. At 4 weeks, 40% laser did have a visible scar on the retina, which suggests it has an effect more closely as threshold than subthreshold therapy. Tissue selectivity for RPE was greater for duty cycles bellow 20% [52]. Furthermore, Lutrull et al. reported a series of 252 patients with macular edema, due to either branch retinal vein occlusion (BRVO) or DME [53]. They compared a 5% duty cycle, versus a 10-15% duty cycle. No damage was found in red free imaging, SD-OCT, fluorescein angiography, ICGA, or infrared imaging in comparison with 8% of patients who underwent laser with 10-15% duty cycle. Subthreshold minimal intensity photocoagulation protocols are therefore designed to minimize tissue damage, while producing only subthreshold thermal effects on the RPE, with an effect that is sustained after treatment in time. Several criteria are therefore implemented for this to be accomplished [51]. There should be an axial confinement of thermal rise in temperature in the area surrounding the laser exposure area, a controlled temperature gradient that minimizes elevated temperatures and thus minimizing lethal heat transfer to the neurosensory retina, and an increase in the tolerance of the chorioretinal tissue to elevated temperatures, inducing a cytoprotective thermal preconditioning making the tissues more resistant to heat damage.

Biological Effect

Gene expression up-regulation is known to have an important role in both angiogenesis and capillary leakage, which are hallmarks of macular and retinal diseases [54]. Laser photocoagulation has shown to regulate the expression of these proteins [55]. After a laser induced lesion, there is a migration of stromal bone marrow derived cells in the treatment area, mediated mainly by stromal cell-derived factor-1 (SDF-1). SDF-1 is produced normally in the RPE cells. It is a chemokine which is involved in the recruitment of hematopoietic cells stem cells into the retinal tissues. SDF-1 therefore is known to be present in a damaged retina, although it's role concerning ocular neovascularization has not been fully understood [55] [56] [57]. Studies show that after a laser burn is made, there is a transient up-regulation of SDF-1 in the first 12 hours after laser treatment, and at two and four weeks, it is virtually undetectable, findings also shown with micropulse laser [52] [58]. A rise in vascular endothelial growth factor (VEGF) was also reported by Yu et al. in the first 12 hours after micropulse subthreshold laser treatment, which tended to fade away within the first three days, with the exception of threshold laser lesions. No levels of insulin-like growth factor (IGF-1) where found after laser treatment [52]. VEGF and IGF-1 have been shown to induce the up regulation for the alpha chemokine receptor for SDF-1 (CXCR4), which may derive in SDF-1 induced angiogenesis [56]. Other factors known to induce vascular proliferation such as transforming growth factor beta II (TGF-βII) have been shown to decrease after both conventional and micropulse laser therapy [59] [60]. The fact that after subthreshold laser treatment, there is little to no up-regulation of these factors proves to be important in reducing the possibilities for angiogenic or neovascularization related complications by laser induced ischemia or damage to the retinal tissues. This is the principle behind macular tissue sparing techniques.

RESULTS

Several studies have shown that patients with CSCR may benefit from conventional laser therapy photocoagulation to the leakage site in order to speed up the recovery times. Nevertheless, several complications associated with laser induced lesions have also been described, especially when the leakage site is located near or in the juxtafoveal and foveal areas. Photodynamic therapy (PDT) has been then used to treat these centrally located cases, although complications have been described with this treatment. The emergence of micropulse therapy has come to address these difficulties. The majority of studies and reports involve 810nm laser, although in recent times, both 532nm and 577nm are being increasingly studied. Initial results have been promising, Bandello et al. first proposed micropulse laser therapy for CSCR in 2003 in a pilot study, in which a small series of cases of CSCR were treated with subthreshold 810nm laser with good results. Since then, subthreshold laser therapy for chronic or recurrent cases has been mostly studied [61]. Cases with a point source leakage tend to have a more favorable response, although diffuse cases still have less than desired results [62].

VISUAL ACUITY

Acute CSCR

Few studies report cases treated before 6 months. Treatment in acute cases has been mostly reserved for patients with an occupational or visual urgency to promptly regain their vision [17]. Conventional laser therapy has been shown to hasten visual recovery in these patients, although with little effect on final BCVA. In recent times, micropulse subthreshold laser therapy has been utilized as relatively new treatment option. Gupta et al. reported in 2009 two cases of patients treated after a one-month history of symptoms [63]. In both cases, initial visual acuity was 20/120. Both cases underwent subthreshold micropulse laser therapy with 810nm wavelength diode laser. The first case presented with complete resolution of symptoms within the first two months, with no recurrence at 12 months follow up and a final visual acuity of 20/25. The second case had an extrafoveal point leak, and after treatment, symptoms resolved within 3 months, with a recurrence at 9 months and a final visual acuity of 20/40. Improvement in visual acuity and contrast sensitivity has been also reported by Behnia et al. with subthreshold argon laser [64]. They reported improvement in mean BCVA of 0.26 to 0.03 in acute cases under one month, an improvement statistically significantly greater than the control group. Nevertheless, the majority of studies show that although there is a more rapid visual recovery, there is little effect on the final visual acuity of patients. Contrast sensitivity did prove to be better in patients treated with subthreshold laser therapy, possibly due to the lack of damage to the neurosensory retina with this treatment [31] [64]. The benefit in final visual acuity seem to not differ between laser and observation groups, although the added benefit of better contrast sensitivity could turn out to be a significant factor for treating these patients [31] [64]. Further studies are currently in place involving a larger study population for these cases [65].

Chronic CSCR

Laser therapy has been mostly utilized in the treatment of chronic or non-resolving cases. Most studies utilize 810nm lasers, although in recent times, 577nm laser therapy has been on the rise. Ricci et al. published a small series of prospective interventional cases, with an average of 6.5 months of persistent symptoms and subretinal fluid, with ICG guided subthreshold 810nm micropulse laser therapy [66] [82]. Mean visual acuity at 12-month follow-up improved on 0.19 logMAR on average ($p < 0.05$), with resolution or improvement of the symptoms in all the cases. Chen et al. reported another case series, with patients with persistent CSCR for more than four months, and a mean follow-up of 14 months. In this prospective, non-comparative case series, mean BVCA improved from 0.348 logMAR to 0.124 logMAR, with a gain of visual acuity of 3 lines or more in 15 eyes (57.7%), and a gain of between 1 and 3 lines in 6 eyes (23.1%). Recent studies have been consistent with these findings. In another case series, Lanzetta et al. published the results of treatment in patients with persistent CSCR over three months [67]. Mean visual acuity was 20/32 before treatment, which improved to 20/25 at the end of the follow-up period. These findings are consistent with more recent reports [66] [67] [68].

In the case of 577nm, similar results have been found [50] [69] [70] [71]. Kim et al. reported a retrospective case series, with a baseline BCVA of 0.21 logMAR, which improved to 0.055 logMAR at three-months follow-up, and 0.035 logMAR at final follow-up period [70]. Similarly, Roisman et al. reported a series of 15 patients treated with the 577nm laser [50]. Comparable results have been obtained on Hispanic populations, where Arias et al. reported in a series of cases, an improvement of a mean 0.8 logMAR to a 0.15 logMAR visual acuity at final follow-up [71]. Larger, prospective interventional studies are needed to confirm and replicate these findings, since there is a lack of such type of investigations, in order to effectively assess the therapeutic effect of subthreshold micropulsed diode laser therapy.

Central Macular Thickness

Acute CSCR

Very few studies address the treatment in acute CSCR, and to our knowledge, no large number of cases have been reported who received subthreshold micropulsed laser therapy. Series of cases reported a more rapid and complete reabsorption of the subretinal fluid although recurrences have been seen. Mean CMT has been seen to be significantly lower when acute CSCR is treated with both PDT and conventional laser therapy when compared to a treatment group [9] [72]. Theoretically, the same effect should be obtained with micropulsed laser therapy, seen as an improvement in the

BCVA seen in the cases reported up to date [63] [64]. Further studies are required to determine the effectiveness to reduce mean CMT in acute patients.

Chronic CSCR

Mean CMT has been seen to decrease with the use of the micropulse diode laser therapy, even with the use of different wavelengths [50] [62] [66] [67] [68] [69] [70] [71] (Figure 1). When compared to an observational approach, laser therapy improves mean CMT in comparison. The decrease in CMT is dependent on the pre-treatment CMT; the greater the mean CMT, more potential for reabsorption there will be [73]. This was seen in the study by Kretz et al., where the observation group had a greater decrease in CMT than the laser treatment group, partly influenced by the baseline mean CMT in these patients. Kim JY et al. reported an improvement after treatment at three months of 99.5μm, which remained so at six months follow-up. CMT has been seen to improve more rapidly in the micropulsed laser treated eyes, especially in the first 3 months after treatment, although the results seem to be comparable at 12 months [70]. This suggests that the effect of subthreshold laser therapy promotes a more rapid anatomical improvement, although has little influence over the final long term results, findings seen also with conventional laser therapy [8] [9] [24]. Further investigations with greater study populations are necessary to study the short and long term effect of this treatment.

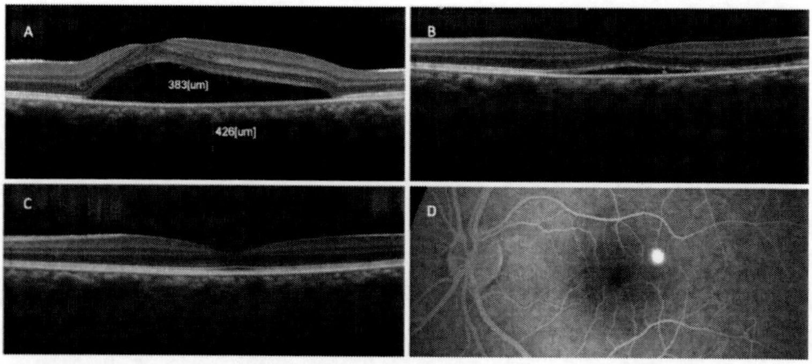

Figure 1. 27yo male with CSCR follow-up after 577nm subthreshold micropulsed diode laser therapy in left eye. A) 2 month history of symptoms. B) 1 month follow-up. C) 1 year follow-up. No disruption in RPE seen. D) Point leakage on fluorescein angiography. Photo courtesy of Manrique Ortiz, MD.

SUBTHRESHOLD LASER THERAPY AND PDT

Photodynamic therapy has been one of the preferred treatment options in recent times to treat CSCR, both acute and chronic, when lesions are found in the foveal or juxtafoveal area, as well as in diffuse CSCR [74] [75] [76] [77]. Mean CMT and BCVA have been seen to improve with PDT, although complications have been reported associated with this therapy. It has been reported that up to 45% of patients treated with PDT have photoreceptor disruption optical coherence tomography (OCT) scans, whether or not this causes a visual deficit is still up to investigation [77] [77]. Decreased macular sensitivity has also been reported in patients treated with PDT when compared to normal fellow eyes [76]. Kretz et al. reported a trial comparing micropulse photocoagulation versus PDT against an observation group, in patients with at least 3 months of subretinal fluid present on OCT [73]. They reported no changes after treatment in the RPE, as there were no significant changes in hyper or hypoautofluorescent lesions on Autofluorescence imaging, either in the laser or the PDT groups. Both treatment groups showed a significant reduction in leakage activity, compared to the control group, with 60-67% of patients showing improvement, against 37.5%. Mean CMT improved by 69.7μm in the laser group, 109.8μm in the PDT group, and 89μm in the control group, largely influenced by the pre-treatment CMT. The number of Early Treatment Diabetic Retinopathy (EDTRS) letters gained were +6.7, +8.5 and +1.5 respectively. The difference between both treatment groups was not statistically significant. They concluded that both treatments resulted in reduced leakage and better BCVA in patients treated with CSCR.

Subthreshold micropulsed laser has also been studied in patients who had received prior treatment with PDT. Breukink et al. evaluated the outcome of patients who underwent two PDT treatments followed by low intensity – high density subthreshold micropulsed 810nm laser therapy [78]. Twelve eyes out of 59 persisted with subretinal fluid after two half dose PDT interventions. Out of these, ten received laser treatment. They reported an 80% reabsorption of the subretinal fluid in these patients, with a mean follow-up of 73 weeks. Mean BVCA improved from 0.28 logMAR to 0.16 logMAR of all eyes, with the most statistically significant improvement after the first treatment. The concluded that with this protocol, there is an anatomical 80% success rate.

SUBTHRESHOLD LASER THERAPY AND ANTI-VEGF

Studies using anti-VEGF agents as treatment for CSCR have been reported in the literature. Even though there have been reports of cases where the use of these agents, mostly bevacizumab, have shown a decrease in the subfoveal CMT in these patients, in the long term the use of them have proven no useful benefits in the treatment of CSCR [32] [79] [80] [67, 68, 69]. The same conclusion is found when comparing ranibizumab with photodynamic therapy [81] [70]. Koss et al. compared 577nm subthreshold laser therapy against bevacizumab and a control group [72] [71]. At ten months' follow-up, 60% of patients treated with bevacizumab had persistent leakage, compared to a 12.5% in the laser therapy group, and 90% in the control group. Mean CMT had the greatest decrease in the laser group, with a decrease of 94 μm, compared to 38μm in the bevacizumab group, and zero in the control group. Mean BVCA improved by six EDTRS letters, decreased by one, and two respectively. Retreatment was required in 43.75% of cases in the laser group, and in 50% of the bevacizumab cases. They also found a larger improvement in the mean perimetric deficit on laser treated patients against the patients who received the anti-VEGF agent. They concluded that 577 subthreshold laser therapy was superior to bevacizumab in the treatment of CSCR.

CHALLENGES WITH MICROPULSE LASER THERAPY

One of the major challenges in subthreshold micropulse laser is the ability to titrate the laser power. Due to the lack of a visible laser lesion to be able to titrate and have a feedback on the energy delivery on the retina to achieve the desirable effect. The possibility, therefore, of treating already treated area is greater with a difficult to determine intensity, increasing the risk for choroidal neovascularization. In addition to this, the fact that the exact mechanisms involving the therapeutic effect of laser therapy are not well understood, it makes it difficult to know when the therapeutic effect will be achieved. The fact that conventional laser has similar therapeutic effects as micropulse laser, the targeting of the RPE seems to be the determining factor. Therefore, some authors have suggested that decreasing the delivery power of conventional laser therapy could have similar therapeutic results [82] [83]. On the contrary, the little to none scarring of the retina and choroid with micropulse laser allows for a more confluent therapy and subsequent retreatment of the already treated areas. Furthermore, micropulse allows for a better control of the irradiance and photothermal effect delivered on the retina. Future challenges include the establishment of treatment protocols and parameters, for several approaches and techniques have been described.

SAFETY PROFILE AND ADVERSE EFFECTS

Certain adverse effects with conventional laser therapy have been described. Amongst the most common ones are decreased visual acuity, visual field defects, decreased color vision, decreased night vision, decreased contrast sensitivity, and pain [84]. Serious complications have been reported, although uncommon. Choroidal neovascularization, hemorrhages, epiretinal fibrosis are of the few adverse effects described in the literature [8] [16] [28]. Micropulsed subthreshold diode laser has come to decrease these complications. Tissue sparing effects of this laser technique has been associated with very few complications reported [53]. When treatment is applied in a low-intensity/high density manner, no changes in the RPE have been detected either in fluorescein angiography, ICGA, red free, infrared, or autofluorenscence imaging [66] [69]. Microperimetry evaluation of treated patients has shown on the contrary, improvement with micropulsed subthreshold laser treatment [85]. A case of increased central retina edema after treatment of CSCR with subthreshold micropulsed diode laser was reported by Gawęcki [86]. Laser power was titrated to 50% of threshold, nevertheless, in fundus autofluorescence, a thermal reaction was seen on the RPE as hyperautofluorescent spots where laser had been applied, followed by an increase in CMT. Retina edema resolved after topical bromfenac and a single treatment of intravitreal bevacizumab. Overall, treatment with subthreshold laser therapy has been shown to produce close to no retinal damage, although further studies must be undertaken to evaluate possible long-term effects on the retinal tissue and RPE.

CONCLUSION

The introduction of infrared subthreshold micropulsed laser therapy, followed by green and yellow laser, has given a new insight in the pathophysiology of CSCR and how laser therapy works. Since the first lasers were used to treat retinovascular and macular diseases, an important advance has been achieved with the introduction of the tissue sparing treatment options. In certain cases of CSCR, the use of this novel treatment can prove to have important benefits for the patients. The possibility to treat foveal or juxtafoveal focal leakage points with minimal risk for damage to the retinal tissues has come to allow treatment of cases in which laser therapy was not an option. This has come to reduce the possibility of adverse effects due to treatment. Laser delivery has proven to be most effective when a low-intensity/high-density approach is applied. The non-visible lesions produced by this therapy poses the challenge to titrate the power correctly in a manner that it produces the required therapeutic effect, without producing a more than desired delivery of energy to the tissues, as well as the treatment of areas previously treated. Most studies to date consist of retrospective, series of cases which require a greater significance in order to provide a larger insight in how the laser works and should be delivered. Laser power titration protocols warrant more studies to effectively deliver the required energy for a therapeutic effect, and reduce risk for complications. Further investigations are needed in order to establish appropriate practice guidelines for the treatment of macular diseases.

References

[1] Yannuzzi, LA. Type-A behavior and central serous chorioretinopathy. *Retina [Internet].*, 1987 [cited 2016 Jul 19], 7(2), 111–31. Available from: http://www.ncbi.nlm.nih.gov/pubmed/3306853.

[2] Von Graefe, A. Ueber centrale recidivierende retinitis. *Graefes Arch Clin Exp Ophthalmol.*, 1866, 12, 211–5.

[3] Gass, JD. Pathogenesis of disciform detachment of the neuroepithelium. *Am J Ophthalmol [Internet].*, 1967 Mar [cited 2016 Jul 19], 63(3), Suppl, 1–139. Available from: http:// www.ncbi.nlm.nih.gov/ pubmed/ 6019308.

[4] Wang, M; Munch, IC; Hasler, PW; Prünte, C; Larsen, M. Central serous chorioretinopathy. *Acta Ophthalmol* [*Internet*]., 2008 Mar [cited 2016 Jul 19], 86(2), 126–45. Available from: http:// www.ncbi.nlm.nih.gov/ pubmed/17662099.

[5] Gilbert, CM; Owens, SL; Smith, PD; Fine, SL. Long-term follow-up of central serous chorioretinopathy. *Br J Ophthalmol* [*Internet*]. 1984 Nov [cited 2016 Jul 19], 68(11), 815–20. Available from: http:// www.ncbi. nlm.nih.gov/pubmed/6541945.

[6] Loo, RH; Scott, IU; Flynn, HW; Gass, JDM; Murray, TG; Lewis, M Lou; et al. Factors associated with reduced visual acuity during long-term follow-up of patients with idiopathic central serous chorioretinopathy. *Retina* [*Internet*]., 2002 Feb [cited 2016 Jul 19], 22(1), 19–24. Available from: http:// www.ncbi.nlm.nih.gov/ pubmed/ 11884873.

[7] Bujarborua, D. Long-term follow-up of idiopathic central serous chorioretinopathy without laser. *Acta Ophthalmol Scand* [*Internet*]., 2001 Aug [cited 2016 Jul 19], 79(4), 417–21. Available from: http:// doi.wiley.com/10.1034/j.1600-0420.2001.079004417.x.

[8] Landers, MB; Shaw, HE; Anderson, WB; Sinyai, AJ. Argon laser treatment of central serous chorioretinopathy. *Ann Ophthalmol* [*Internet*]., 1977 Dec [cited 2016 Jul 19], 9(12), 1567–72. Available from: http://www.ncbi.nlm.nih.gov/pubmed/564655.

[9] Leaver, P; Williams, C. Argon laser photocoagulation in the treatment of central serous retinopathy. *Br J Ophthalmol* [*Internet*]., 1979 Oct [cited 2016 Jul 19], 63(10), 674–7. Available from: http:// www.ncbi.nlm.nih. gov/pubmed/574397.

[10] Dinc, UA; Tatlipinar, S; Yenerel, M; Görgün, E; Ciftci, F. Fundus autofluorescence in acute and chronic central serous chorioretinopathy. *Clin Exp Optom* [*Internet*]., 2011 Sep [cited 2016 Jul 19], 94(5), 452–7. Available from: http://www.ncbi.nlm.nih.gov/pubmed/21480989.

[11] Chan, SY; Wang, Q; Wei, W Bin; Jonas, JB. Optical Coherence Tomographic Angiography In Central Serous Chorioretinopathy. *Retina [Internet]*., 2016 May 9 [Cited 2016 Jul 19], 1. Available From: http:// www.ncbi.nlm.nih.gov/pubmed/27164548.

[12] Marshall, J. Lasers in Ophthalmology: The Basic Principles. *Eye*.. 1988, 2, 98–112.

[13] Novak, MA; Singerman, LJ; Rice, TA. Krypton and argon laser photocoagulation for central serous chorioretinopathy. *Retina [Internet]*., 1987 [cited 2016 Jul 19], 7(3), 162–9. Available from: http://www.ncbi.nlm.nih.gov/pubmed/3423431.

[14] Roseman, RL; Olk, RJ. Grid laser photocoagulation for atypical central serous chorioretinopathy. *Ophthalmic Surg [Internet]*., 1988 Nov [cited 2016 Jul 19], 19(11), 786–91. Available from: http:// www.ncbi.nlm.nih. gov/pubmed/3222040.

[15] Fong, DS; Girach, A; Boney, A. Visual side effects of successful scatter laser photocoagulation surgery for proliferative diabetic retinopathy: a literature review. *Retina [Internet]*., 2007 Sep [cited 2016 Jul 19], 27(7),

816–24. Available from: http:// www.ncbi.nlm.nih.gov/ pubmed/ 17891003.

[16] Berger, AR; Boniuk, I. Bilateral subretinal neovascularization after focal argon laser photocoagulation for diabetic macular edema. *Am J Ophthalmol [Internet]*., 1989 Jul 15 [cited 2016 Jul 19], 108(1), 88–90. Available from: http://www.ncbi.nlm.nih.gov/pubmed/2473649.

[17] Schubert, H; Atebara, N; Kaiser, R; Martidis, A; McCannel, C; Zacks, D; et al. Choroidal Disease. In: Schubert H, editor. Basic Clinical and Science Course. 2012th–3rd ed. *San Francisco: American Academy of Ophthalmology*, 2012.

[18] L'Esperance, FA; Meyer-Schwickerath, G; Guerry, D; Wiesinger, H; Pischel, DK; Meyer-Schwickerath, G; Guerry, D; III et al. Clinical Comparison of Xenon-Arc and Laser Photocoagulation of Retinal Lesions. *Arch Ophthalmol [Internet]*., 1966 Jan 1 [cited 2016 Jul 19], 75(1), 61–7. Available from: http:// archopht.jamanetwork.com/ article. aspx?articleid=628261.

[19] Plumb, AP; Swan, AV; Chignell, AH; Shilling, JS. A comparative trial of xenon arc and argon laser photocoagulation in the treatment of proliferative diabetic retinopathy. *Br J Ophthalmol [Internet]*., 1982 Apr [cited 2016 Jul 19], 66(4), 213–8. Available from: http:// www.ncbi. nlm.nih.gov/pubmed/6175340.

[20] Littell, A. Photocoagulation treatment of proliferative diabetic retinopathy. Clinical application of Diabetic Retinopathy Study (DRS) findings, DRS Report Number 8. The Diabetic Retinopathy Study Research Group. *Ophthalmology [Internet]*., 1981 Jul [cited 2016 Jul 19], 88(7), 583–600. Available from: http:// linkinghub.elsevier.com/ retrieve/pii/S0161642081349781.

[21] Kapany, Ns; Peppers, Na; Zweng, Hc; Flocks, M. Retinal Photocoagulation By Lasers. *Nature [Internet]*., 1963 Jul 13 [cited 2016 Jul 19], 199, 146–9. Available from: http:// www.ncbi.nlm.nih.gov/ pubmed/14043179.

[22] Noyori, Ks; Campbell, Jc; Rittler, Mc; Koester, C; Guerry, DI; Ham, WTJ; et al. Ocular Thermal Effects Produced by Photocoagulation. *Arch Ophthalmol [Internet]*., 1963 Dec 1 [cited 2016 Jul 19], 70(6), 817–22. Available from: http:// archopht.jamanetwork.com/ article.aspx? articleid =627410.

[23] Watzke, RC; Burton, TC; Leaverton, PE. Ruby laser photocoagulation therapy of central serous retinopathy. I. A controlled clinical study. II. Factors affecting prognosis. *Trans Am Acad Ophthalmol Otolaryngol*

[Internet]., 1974 [cited 2016 Jul 19], 78(2), OP205–11. Available from: http://www.ncbi.nlm.nih.gov/pubmed/4856872.

[24] Makabe, R. [Krypton and argon laser coagulation in chorioretinitis centralis serosa]. *Klin Monatsblätter für Augenheilkd [Internet].*, 1987 Jun [cited 2016 Jul 19], 190(6), 489–90. Available from: http:// www.ncbi.nlm.nih.gov/pubmed/3626406.

[25] Slusher, MM. Krypton red laser photocoagulation in selected cases of central serous chorioretinopathy. *Retina [Internet].*, 1986 [cited 2016 Jul 19], 6(2), 81–4. Available from: http:// www.ncbi.nlm.nih.gov/ pubmed/ 3749625.

[26] Grabowski, WM; Decker, WL; Annesley, WH; Group, MPS; Bird, A; Grey, R; et al. Complications of Krypton Red Laser Photocoagulation to Subretinal Neovascular Membranes. *Ophthalmology [Internet].*, 1984 Dec [cited 2016 Jul 19], 91(12), 1587–91. Available from: http:// linkinghub.elsevier.com/retrieve/pii/S0161642084341148.

[27] Gole, GA. Massive choroidal haemorrhage as a complication of krypton red laser photocoagulation for disciform degeneration. *Aust N Z J Ophthalmol [Internet].*, 1985 Feb [cited 2016 Jul 19], 13(1), 37–8. Available from: http://www.ncbi.nlm.nih.gov/pubmed/2409995.

[28] Schatz, H; Yannuzzi, LA; Gitter, KA. Subretinal neovascularization following argon laser photocoagulation treatment for central serous chorioretinopathy: complication or misdiagnosis? 1975. *Retina [Internet].*, 2012 Feb [cited 2016 Jul 19], 32 Suppl 1, OP893–906. Available from: http://www.ncbi.nlm.nih.gov/pubmed/22379619.

[29] Guyer, DR; Yannuzzi, LA; Slakter, JS; Sorenson, JA; Ho, A; Orlock, D. Digital indocyanine green videoangiography of central serous chorioretinopathy. *Arch Ophthalmol (Chicago, Ill 1960) [Internet].*, 1994 Aug [cited 2016 Jul 19], 112(8), 1057–62. Available from: http://www.ncbi.nlm.nih.gov/pubmed/8053819.

[30] Mosier, MA; Champion, J; Liaw, LH; Berns, MW. Retinal effects of the frequency-doubled (532 nm) YAG laser: histopathological comparison with argon laser. *Lasers Surg Med [Internet].*, 1985 [cited 2016 Jul 19], 5(4), 377–404. Available from: http:// www.ncbi.nlm.nih.gov/ pubmed/ 3839881.

[31] Klatt, C; Saeger, M; Oppermann, T; Pörksen, E; Treumer, F; Hillenkamp, J; et al. Selective retina therapy for acute central serous chorioretinopathy. *Br J Ophthalmol [Internet].*, 2011 Jan [cited 2016 Jul 19], 95(1) 83–8. Available from: http://www.ncbi.nlm.nih.gov/ pubmed/ 20554506.

[32] Kim, DY; Joe, SG; Yang, SJ; Lee, JY; Kim, JG; Yoon, YH; et al. The Association between Choroidal Thickness Variations and Response to Intravitreal Bevacizumab in Central Serous Chorioretinopathy. *Korean J Ophthalmol [Internet]*., 2015 [cited 2016 Jul 19], 29(3), 160. Available from: http:// synapse.koreamed.org/ DOIx.php?id=10.3341/ kjo.2015. 29.3.160.

[33] Sturm, V; Schwartz, R; Richard, G. Early laser photocoagulation in Central Serous Chorioretinopathy. *Invest Ophthalmol Vis Sci*., 2004, 45(13), 532–532.

[34] Verma, L; Sinha, R; Venkatesh, P; Tewari, H; Maumenee, A; Scheider, A; et al. Comparative evaluation of diode laser versus argon laser photocoagulation in patients with central serous retinopathy: A pilot, randomized controlled trial [ISRCTN84128484]. *BMC Ophthalmol [Internet]*., 2004 Dec 29 [cited 2016 Jul 19]; 4(1):15. Available from: http://bmcophthalmol.biomedcentral.com/articles/10.1186/1471-2415-4-15.

[35] Mainster, MA; Ho, PC; Mainster, KJ. Argon and Krypton Laser Photocoagulators. *Ophthalmology [Internet]*., 1983 Jan [cited 2016 Jul 19], 90(9), 48–54. Available from: http:// linkinghub.elsevier.com/ retrieve/pii/S0161642083344225.

[36] Mainster, MA; Ho, PC; Mainster, KJ; Mainster, M; Sliney, D; Belcher, C; et al. Nd:YAG Laser Photodisruptors. *Ophthalmology [Internet]*., 1983 Jan [cited 2016 Jul 19], 90(9), 45. Available from: http:// linkinghub.elsevier.com/retrieve/pii/S0161642083344201.

[37] Balles, MW; Puliafito, CA. Semiconductor diode lasers: a new laser light source in ophthalmology. *Int Ophthalmol Clin [Internet]*., 1990 [cited 2016 Jul 19], 30(2), 77–83. Available from: http:// www.ncbi.nlm. nih.gov/pubmed/2185176.

[38] Mainster, MA. Wavelength Selection in Macular Photocoagulation. *Ophthalmology [Internet]*., 1986 Jul [cited 2016 Jul 19], 93(7), 952–8. Available from: http://linkinghub.elsevier.com/retrieve/pii/S01616 42086336376.

[39] Daruich, A; Matet, A; Dirani, A; Bousquet, E; Zhao, M; Farman, N; et al. Central serous chorioretinopathy: Recent findings and new physiopathology hypothesis. *Prog Retin Eye Res [Internet]*., 2015 Sep, 48, 82–118. Available from: http:// www.sciencedirect.com/ science/ article/pii/S1350946215000336.

[40] Trempe, CL; Mainster, MA; Pomerantzeff, O; Avila, MP; Jalkh, AE; Weiter, JJ; et al. Macular Photocoagulation. *Ophthalmology [Internet]*.,

1982 Jul [cited 2016 Jul 19], 89(7), 721–8. Available from: http://linkinghub.elsevier.com/retrieve/pii/S0161642082347351.

[41] Lanzetta, P; Dorin, G; Pirracchio, A; Bandello, F. Theoretical bases of non-ophthalmoscopically visible endpoint photocoagulation. *Semin Ophthalmol [Internet].*, 2001 Mar [cited 2016 Jul 19], 16(1), 8–11. Available from: http://www.ncbi.nlm.nih.gov/pubmed/15487692.

[42] Mainster, MA. Decreasing retinal photocoagulation damage: principles and techniques. *Semin Ophthalmol [Internet].*, 1999 Dec [cited 2016 Jul 19], 14(4), 200–9. Available from: http:// www.ncbi.nlm.nih.gov/ pubmed/10758220.

[43] Dorin, G. Subthreshold and micropulse diode laser photocoagulation. *Semin Ophthalmol [Internet].*, 2003 Sep [cited 2016 Jul 19], 18(3), 147–53. Available from: http://www.ncbi.nlm.nih.gov/pubmed/15513476.

[44] Brancato, R; Pratesi, R; Leoni, G; Trabucchi, G; Vanni, U. Histopathology of diode and argon laser lesions in rabbit retina. A comparative study. *Invest Ophthalmol Vis Sci [Internet].*, 1989 Jul [cited 2016 Jul 19], 30(7), 1504–10. Available from: http:// www.ncbi.nlm. nih.gov/pubmed/2744993.

[45] Lavinsky, D; Sramek, C; Wang, J; Huie, P; Dalal, R; Mandel, Y; et al. Subvisible retinal laser therapy: titration algorithm and tissue response. *Retina [Internet].*, 2014 Jan [cited 2016 Jul 19], 34(1), 87–97. Available from: http://www.ncbi.nlm.nih.gov/pubmed/23873164.

[46] Kim, SY; Sanislo, SR; Dalal, R; et al. The selective effect of micropulse diode laser upon the retina. *Invest Ophthalmol Vis Sci.*, 1996, 37(3), S779.

[47] Pollack, JS; Kim, JE; Pulido, JS; Burke, JMTHMJWB; et al. Tissue Effects of Subclinical Diode Laser Treatment of the Retina. *Arch Ophthalmol [Internet].*, 1998 Dec 1 [cited 2016 Jul 19], 116(12), 1633. Available from: http:// archopht.jamanetwork.com/ article.aspx? doi=10.1001/archopht.116.12.1633.

[48] Lavinsky, D; Cardillo, JA; Melo, LAS; Dare, A; Farah, ME; Belfort, R. Randomized clinical trial evaluating mETDRS versus normal or high-density micropulse photocoagulation for diabetic macular edema. *Invest Ophthalmol Vis Sci [Internet].*, 2011 Jun [cited 2016 Jul 19], 52(7), 4314–23. Available from: http:// www.ncbi.nlm.nih.gov/ pubmed/21345996.

[49] Lavinsky, D; Palanker, D. Nondamaging photothermal therapy for the retina: initial clinical experience with chronic central serous retinopathy.

Retina [Internet]., 2015 Feb [cited 2016 Jul 19], 35(2), 213–22. Available from: http://www.ncbi.nlm.nih.gov/pubmed/25158944.

[50] Kim, JY; Park, HS; Kim, SY. Short-term efficacy of subthreshold micropulse yellow laser (577-nm) photocoagulation for chronic central serous chorioretinopathy. *Graefe's Arch Clin Exp Ophthalmol [Internet].*, 2015 Dec 26 [cited 2016 Jul 19], 253(12), 2129–35. Available from: http://link.springer.com/10.1007/s00417-015-2965-7.

[51] Dorin, G. Evolution of retinal laser therapy: minimum intensity photocoagulation (MIP). Can the laser heal the retina without harming it? *Semin Ophthalmol [Internet].*, 2004 [cited 2016 Jul 19], 19(1-2), 62–8. Available from: http://www.ncbi.nlm.nih.gov/pubmed/15590536.

[52] Yu, AK; Merrill, KD; Truong, SN; Forward, KM; Morse, LS; Telander, DG. The Comparative Histologic Effects of Subthreshold 532- and 810-nm Diode Micropulse Laser on the Retina. *Investig Opthalmology Vis Sci [Internet].*, 2013 Mar 27 [cited 2016 Jul 19], 54(3), 2216. Available from: http://www.ncbi.nlm.nih.gov/pubmed/23439599.

[53] Luttrull, JK; Sramek, C; Palanker, D; Spink, CJ; Musch, DC. Long-term safety, high-resolution imaging, and tissue temperature modeling of subvisible diode micropulse photocoagulation for retinovascular macular edema. *Retina [Internet].*, 2012 Feb [cited 2016 Jul 19], 32(2), 375–86. Available from: http://www.ncbi.nlm.nih.gov/pubmed/21971077.

[54] Chen, L; Zhuo, Y; Li, Y; Huang, X; Zhang, J; Li, S; et al. Expression of stromal cell-derived factor-1 in diabetic retinopathy. *Chin Med J (Engl) [Internet].*, 2010 Apr 20 [cited 2016 Jul 19], 123(8), 984–8. Available from: http://www.ncbi.nlm.nih.gov/pubmed/20497701.

[55] Wilson, AS; Hobbs, BG; Shen, WY; Speed, TP; Schmidt, U; Begley, CG; et al. Argon laser photocoagulation-induced modification of gene expression in the retina. Invest Ophthalmol Vis Sci [Internet]. 2003 Apr [cited 2016 Jul 19], 44(4), 1426–34. Available from: http:// www.ncbi.nlm.nih.gov/pubmed/12657576.

[56] Sengupta, N; Afzal, A; Caballero, S; Chang, KH; Shaw, LC; Pang, JJ; et al. Paracrine Modulation of CXCR4 by IGF-1 and VEGF: Implications for Choroidal Neovascularization. *Investig Opthalmology Vis Sci [Internet].*, 2010 May 1 [cited 2016 Jul 19]; 51(5), 2697. Available from: http://www.ncbi.nlm.nih.gov/pubmed/20007826.

[57] Lima e Silva, R; Shen, J; Hackett, SF; Kachi, S; Akiyama, H; Kiuchi, K; et al. The SDF-1/CXCR4 ligand/receptor pair is an important contributor to several types of ocular neovascularization. *FASEB J [Internet].*, 2007

Oct 1 [cited 2016 Jul 19], 21(12), 3219–30. Available from: http://www.fasebj.org/cgi/doi/10.1096/fj.06-7359com.
[58] Lai, P; Li, T; Yang, J; Xie, C; Zhu, X; Xie, H; et al. Upregulation of stromal cell–derived factor 1 (SDF-1) expression in microvasculature endothelial cells in retinal ischemia-reperfusion injury. *Graefe's Arch Clin Exp Ophthalmol [Internet].*, 2008 Dec 16 [cited 2016 Jul 19], 246(12), 1707–13. Available from: http:// www.ncbi.nlm.nih.gov/ pubmed/18709383.
[59] Ruskovic, D; Boulton, M; Ulbig, MW; et al. The effect of micropulsed diode laser on the human RPE *in vivo* and *in vitro*. *Invest Ophthalmol Vis Sci.*, 1997, 38(4), S754.
[60] Stayt, J; Gillies, MC. TGF-b increases permeability of retinal capillary endothelial cell monolayers and is associated with tyrosine phosphorylation of intercellular proteins. *Invest Ophthalmol Vis Sci.*, 1997, 38(4), S791.
[61] Bandello, F; Lanzetta, P; Furlan, F; Polito, A. Non Visible Subthreshold Micropulse Diode Laser Treatment of Idiopathic Central Serous Chorioretinopathy. *A Pilot Study. Invest Ophthalmol Vis Sci.*, 2003, 44(13), 4858–4858.
[62] Chen, SN; Hwang, JF; Tseng, LF; Lin, CJ. Subthreshold diode micropulse photocoagulation for the treatment of chronic central serous chorioretinopathy with juxtafoveal leakage. *Ophthalmology [Internet].*, 2008 Dec [cited 2016 Jul 19], 115(12), 2229–34. Available from: http://www.ncbi.nlm.nih.gov/pubmed/19041477.
[63] Gupta, B; Elagouz, M; McHugh, D; Chong, V; Sivaprasad, S. Micropulse diode laser photocoagulation for central serous chorio-retinopathy. *Clin Experiment Ophthalmol [Internet].*, 2009 Nov [cited 2016 Jul 19], 37(8), 801–5. Available from: http:// doi.wiley.com/ 10.1111/j.1442-9071.2009.02157.x.
[64] Behnia, M; Khabazkhoob, M; Aliakbari, S; Abadi, AE; Hashemi, H; Pourvahidi, P. Improvement in visual acuity and contrast sensitivity in patients with central serous chorioretinopathy after macular subthreshold laser therapy. *Retina [Internet].*, 2013 Feb [cited 2016 Jul 19], 33(2), 324–8. Available from: http://www.ncbi.nlm.nih.gov/pubmed/23314231.
[65] Breukink, MB; Downes, SM; Querques, G; van Dijk, EHC; den Hollander, AI; Blanco-Garavito, R; et al. Comparing half-dose photodynamic therapy with high-density subthreshold micropulse laser treatment in patients with chronic central serous chorioretinopathy (the PLACE trial): study protocol for a randomized controlled trial. *Trials*

[Internet]., 2015 Dec 21 [cited 2016 Jul 19], 16(1), 419. Available from: http://www.trialsjournal.com/content/16/1/419.

[66] Ricci, F; Missiroli, F; Regine, F; Grossi, M; Dorin, G. Indocyanine green enhanced subthreshold diode-laser micropulse photocoagulation treatment of chronic central serous chorioretinopathy. *Graefe's Arch Clin Exp Ophthalmol = Albr von Graefes Arch für Klin und Exp Ophthalmol [Internet].*, 2009 May [cited 2016 Jul 19], 247(5), 597–607. Available from: http://www.ncbi.nlm.nih.gov/pubmed/19089442.

[67] Lanzetta, P; Furlan, F; Morgante, L; Veritti, D; Bandello, F. Nonvisible subthreshold micropulse diode laser (810 nm) treatment of central serous chorioretinopathy. A pilot study. *Eur J Ophthalmol [Internet].*, 2008 [cited 2016 Jul 19], 18(6), 934–40. Available from: http:// www.ncbi.nlm.nih.gov/pubmed/18988165.

[68] Malik, KJ; Sampat, KM; Mansouri, A; Steiner, JN; Glaser, BM. Low-intensity/high-density subthreshold microPulse diode laser for chronic central serous chorioretinopathy. Retina [Internet]. 2015 Mar [cited 2016 Jul 19], 35(3), 532–6. Available from: http:// www.ncbi.nlm.nih.gov/pubmed/25127050.

[69] Luttrull, JK. Low-intensity/high-density subthreshold diode micropulse laser for central serous chorioretinopathy. *Retina [Internet].*, 2016 Mar 3 [cited 2016 Jul 19], Available from: http:// www.ncbi.nlm.nih.gov/pubmed/27206160.

[70] Roisman, L; Magalhães, FP; Lavinsky, D; Moraes, N; Hirai, FE; Cardillo, JA; et al. Micropulse diode laser treatment for chronic central serous chorioretinopathy: a randomized pilot trial. *Ophthalmic Surg Lasers Imaging Retina [Internet].*, 2013 [cited 2016 Jul 19], 44(5), 465–70. Available from: http://www.ncbi.nlm.nih.gov/pubmed/24044709.

[71] Arias, JD; Galvis, V; Barrera, R; et al. Photostimulation subthreshold Pascal laser in the treatment of central serous chorioretinopathy pilot study. *Poster ASRS 2015*. Vienna, 2015.

[72] Koss, MJ; Beger, I; Koch, FH. Subthreshold diode laser micropulse photocoagulation versus intravitreal injections of bevacizumab in the treatment of central serous chorioretinopathy. *Eye (Lond) [Internet].*, 2012 Feb [cited 2016 Jul 19], 26(2), 307–14. Available from: http://www.ncbi.nlm.nih.gov/pubmed/22079961.

[73] Kretz, FTA; Beger, I; Koch, F; Nowomiejska, K; Auffarth, GU; Koss, MJ. Randomized Clinical Trial to Compare Micropulse Photocoagulation Versus Half-dose Verteporfin Photodynamic Therapy in the Treatment of Central Serous Chorioretinopathy. *Ophthalmic Surg*

Lasers Imaging Retina [Internet]., 2015 Sep [cited 2016 Jul 19], 46(8), 837–43. Available from: http:// www.ncbi.nlm.nih.gov/ pubmed/ 26431299.

[74] Chan, WM; Lai, TYY; Lai, RYK; Liu, DTL; Lam, DSC. Half-dose verteporfin photodynamic therapy for acute central serous chorioretinopathy: one-year results of a randomized controlled trial. *Ophthalmology [Internet]*., 2008 Oct [cited 2016 Jul 19], 115(10), 1756–65. Available from: http:// www.ncbi.nlm.nih.gov/ pubmed/ 18538401.

[75] Alkin, Z; Perente, I; Ozkaya, A; Yasa, D; Agca, A; Aygit, ED; et al. Comparison of efficacy between low-fluence and half-dose verteporfin photodynamic therapy for chronic central serous chorioretinopathy. *Clin Ophthalmol [Internet]*., 2014 Apr [cited 2016 Jul 19], Volume 8, 685. Available from: http://www.dovepress.com/comparison-of-efficacy-between-low-fluence-and-half-dose-verteporfin-p-peer-reviewed-article-OPTH.

[76] Sanguansak, T; Pitujaturont, P; Yospaiboon, Y; Sinawat, S; Ratanapakorn, T; Bhoomibunchoo, C. Macular sensitivity after half-dose verteporfin photodynamic therapy in central serous chorioretinopathy. *Clin Ophthalmol [Internet]*., 2015, 9, 2257–61. Available from: http://www.ncbi.nlm.nih.gov/pubmed/26664040.

[77] Ratanasukon, M; Thongthong, Bhurayanontachai P Jirarattanasopa. Photoreceptor disruption in central serous chorioretinopathy treated by half-dose photodynamic therapy. *Clin Ophthalmol [Internet]*., 2013 Jan [cited 2016 Jul 19], Volume 7, 87. Available from: http:// www. dovepress.com/photoreceptor-disruption-in-central-serous-chorioretinopathy-treated-b-peer-reviewed-article-OPTH.

[78] Breukink, MB; Mohr, JK; Ossewaarde-van Norel, A; den Hollander, AI; Keunen, JEE; Hoyng, CB; et al. Half-dose photodynamic therapy followed by diode micropulse laser therapy as treatment for chronic central serous chorioretinopathy: evaluation of a prospective treatment protocol. *Acta Ophthalmol [Internet]*., 2016 Mar 1, 94(2), 187–97. Available from: http://dx.doi.org/10.1111/aos.12938.

[79] Park, SU; Lee, SJ; Kim, M; Levine, R; Brucker, A; Robinson, F; et al. Intravitreal Anti-vascular Endothelial Growth Factor versus Observation in Acute Central Serous Chorioretinopathy: One-year Results. *Korean J Ophthalmol [Internet]*., 2014 [cited 2016 Jul 19], 28(4), 306. Available from: http:// synapse.koreamed.org/ DOIx.php?id=10.3341/ kjo.2014.28. 4.306.

[80] Chung, YR; Seo, EJ; Lew, HM; Lee, KH. Lack of positive effect of intravitreal bevacizumab in central serous chorioretinopathy: meta-analysis and review. *Eye [Internet].*, 2013 Dec, 27(12), 1339–46. Available from: http://dx.doi.org/10.1038/eye.2013.236.

[81] Bae, SH; Heo, JW; Kim, C; Kim, TW; Lee, JY; Song, SJ; et al. A Randomized Pilot Study of Low-Fluence Photodynamic Therapy Versus Intravitreal Ranibizumab for Chronic Central Serous Chorioretinopathy. Am J Ophthalmol [Internet]. 2011 Nov [cited 2016 Jul 19]; 152(5):784–92.e2. Available from: http://linkinghub.elsevier.com/retrieve/pii/S0002939411003199.

[82] Bandello, F; Brancato, R; Menchini, U; Virgili, G; Lanzetta, P; Ferrari, E; et al. Light panretinal photocoagulation (LPRP) versus classic panretinal photocoagulation (CPRP) in proliferative diabetic retinopathy. *Semin Ophthalmol [Internet].*, 2001 Mar [cited 2016 Jul 19], 16(1), 12–8. Available from: http://www.ncbi.nlm.nih.gov/pubmed/15487693.

[83] Cardillo, JA; Lavinsky, DLAS; Melo, J; Dare, A; Castro, L; Costa, RA; et al. Comparison of the Modified Early Treatment Diabetic Retinopathy Study and Normal or High Density Subthreshold Infrared Micro Pulsed Photocoagulation for Diabetic Macular Edema. *Invest Ophthalmol Vis Sci.*, 2008, 49(13), 1566–1566.

[84] Sivaprasad, S; Elagouz, M; McHugh, D; Shona, O; Dorin, G. Micropulsed Diode Laser Therapy: Evolution and Clinical Applications. *Surv Ophthalmol [Internet].*, 2010 Nov 14, 55(6), 516–30. Available from: http://dx.doi.org/10.1016/j.survophthal.2010.02.005.

[85] Yadav, NK; Jayadev, C; Mohan, A; Vijayan, P; Battu, R; Dabir, S; et al. Subthreshold micropulse yellow laser (577 nm) in chronic central serous chorioretinopathy: safety profile and treatment outcome. *Eye (Lond) [Internet].*, 2015 Feb [cited 2016 Jul 19], 29(2), 258–64, quiz 265. Available from: http://www.ncbi.nlm.nih.gov/pubmed/25613846.

[86] Gawęcki, M. Increase in Central Retinal Edema after Subthreshold Diode Micropulse Laser Treatment of Chronic Central Serous Chorioretinopathy. *Case Rep Ophthalmol Med [Internet].*, 2015 [cited 2016 Jul 19], 2015, 813414. Available from: http:// www.ncbi.nlm.nih.gov/pubmed/26180649.

Biographical Sketch

Name: Federico Ortiz
Affiliation: Clinica Oftalmocima, San Jose, Costa Rica
Caja Costarricense del Seguro Social, San Jose, Costa Rica
Education: Universidad de Costa Rica

Name: Juan Carlos Gutierrez-Hernandez
Affiliation: Hospital Clinica Biblica, San Jose, Costa Rica
Caja Costarricense del Seguro Social, San Jose, Costa Rica
Universidad de Costa Rica, San José, Costa Rica.
Education: Universidad de Costa Rica (UCR)
Universidad Nacional Autónoma de México (UNAM)
Universidad de Guadalajara (UDG)
University of Southern California (USC)
Doheny Eye Institute (DEI)
Research and Professional Experience: Retina Research Fellowship 2011-2012
Publications Last 3 Years:

Long-term follow-up of photoreceptor loss and recovery after half-fluence photodynamic therapy for chronic central serous chorioretinopathy. Gutiérrez-Hernández JC, Martínez-Camarillo JC, Sadda SR. Retin Cases Brief Rep. 2015 Spring; 9(2): 109-13. doi: 10.1097/ ICB.0000000000000105. PMID:25383847

Collaborative retrospective macula society study of photodynamic therapy for chronic central serous chorioretinopathy. Lim JI, Glassman AR, Aiello LP, Chakravarthy U, Flaxel CJ, Spaide RF; Macula Society CSC Collaborative Study Group, Research and Education Committee and Website Committee. Ophthalmology. 2014 May; 121(5):1073-8. doi: 10.1016/j.ophtha.2013.11.040. Epub 2014 Jan 16.PMID:24439758

One-Year Feasibility Study of Replenish MicroPump for Intravitreal Drug Delivery: A Pilot Study. Gutiérrez-Hernández JC, Caffey S, Abdallah W, Calvillo P, González R, Shih J, Brennan J, Zimmerman J, Martínez-Camarillo JC, Rodriguez AR, Varma R, Santos A, Sánchez G, Humayun M. Transl Vis Sci Technol. 2014 Jul 1; 3(4): 8. eCollection 2014 May. PMID:25774328

Santos-García A. “El libro Grin de Oftalmología”, ISBN 978-607-9024-30-7, 682 p. Editorial Publicaciones Encuadre, 2014.

Name: Alonso Gutiérrez
Affiliation: Universidad de Costa Rica
Education: Universidad de Costa Rica

In: Central Serous Chorioretinopathy (CSCR)
Editor: Patrick Evans
ISBN: 978-1-53610-806-4

Chapter 4

ALTERNATIVE SYSTEMIC TREATMENTS FOR CENTRAL SEROUS CHORIORETINOPATHY

Alonso Gutiérrez-Guerinoni[1,*], MD, Federico Ortíz-Coto[2], MD and Juan Carlos Gutiérrez-Hernández[3], MD

[1]Department of Ophthalmology, Universidad de Costa Rica, San Jose, Costa Rica

[2]Clinica Oftalmocima, Caja Costarricense del Seguro Social, San Jose, Costa Rica

[3]Hospital Clinica Biblica, Caja Costarricense del Seguro Social, Universidad de Costa Rica, San Jose, Costa Rica

ABSTRACT

There is no fully effective treatment for central serous chorioretinopathy, therefore investigators have proposed and explored a series of interventional alternatives. These alternatives include local and systemic oral therapy.

The pathophysiology of the disease is still not thoroughly understood and the exact role of corticosteroids is unclear. Several hypotheses have been suggested on the physiopathology of this disease. However, recent

[*] Corresponding author: dralonsogutierrez@gmail.com.

research has demonstrated the importance of glucocorticoids and mineralocorticoids. Animal models have proved influence of these hormones on choroidal permeability, leading to usage of antiglucocorticoid medications as treatment. Pilot studies have demonstrated certain efficiency clinically with improvements in visual acuity and macular morphology. Results are varied but antiglucocorticoid medication seems to be a promising alternative.

Excessive epinephrine may affect the retina through beta-adrenergic receptors on the retinal pigment epithelium. Activation of these receptors has been shown to produce a change in cyclic adenosine monophosphate concentration, affecting retinal pigment epithelium's electrical activity. Epinephrine has also been shown to induce apoptosis in retinal pigment epithelium cells *in vitro*, leading to the proposal of propranolol and other beta-blockers as alternative therapy. Results have been mixed on the use of beta-blockers making other alternatives more promising.

The choroidal vasculature has been the base of mineralocorticoid antagonist therapy such as spironolactone, eplerenone, mifepristone and ketoconazole, or the 5α-reductase inhibiting drug finasteride.

Finasteride has been used due to its antiandrogenic effects but due to its side effects could have limitations in clinical use for CSC.

Reduction of the expression of steroid receptors has also been proposed as a target with therapy through low doses of methotrexate and melatonin but further research is necessary.

Aspiring has also been used for its effects on coagulation and plasminogen activator inhibitor. Although further investigation is required it has been found to improve visual acuity.

Rifampin is one of the most widely used and investigated oral treatments. Its properties induce cytochrome P450 therefore accelerating steroid metabolism, leading to a decrease in plasma steroids. Such decrease has been demonstrated on both exogenous and endogenous steroids, driving many case report series with promising results as a therapeutic alternative.

Recent data has demonstrated correlation between Helicobacter pylori infection and CSC. Studies have used treatment against this bacillus on patients with CSC, however results have been mixed.

There are many publications with these unconventional options, nevertheless most of them are small number case series, and require longer follow up and a larger number of cases. Randomized studies need to be published in order to understand the long-term efficiency, recurrences and safety of these non-invasive alternatives.

Keywords: central serous chorioretinopathy, systemic, oral, alternative, metipranolol, propranolol, spirolactone, eplerenone, methotrexate, mifepristone, ketoconazole, rifampin, melatonin, finasteride, aspirin, Helicobacter pylori

INTRODUCTION

Central serous chorioretinopathy (CSC) is an idiopathic condition typically affecting men from 20 to 50 years of age [1]. The annual incidence is 9.9 per 100,000 individuals for men and 1.7 for women, pinpointing 6-time higher incidence in men than in women [2]. CSC is characterized by accumulation of subretinal fluid causing well-circumscribed serous retinal detachments. The natural course of this condition is usually self-limited with spontaneous resolution in most cases. A fraction of these cases persist or recur leading to long-term visual impairments. The chronic form, known as diffuse retinal epitheliopathy, is usually bilateral with widespread retinal pigment epithelium alterations and varying intraretinal cysts. To this date, the pathogenesis of the disease is still not completely understood, however investigations show the choroid to be the primary site of dysfunction.

Recent studies have put mineralocorticoid antagonism in the spotlight although the exact role they play is unclear; several studies have had success using mineralocorticoid antagonists. Although only proven in animal models, Zhao et al. [3], induced choroidal enlargement through intravitreous injections of high doses of glucocorticoids.

The retina and the choroid have mineralocorticoid receptors (MR), which can be activated by aldosterone or cortisol; continual activation by cortisol on MR is prevented by 11-beta hydroxysteroid dehydrogenase type 2 [4]. This enzyme is found in tissue sensitive to mineralocorticoids, proving that the retina and the choroid are receptive of these hormones. Aldosterone induces an endothelial potassium channel, KCa2.3 activating calcium dependent channels to cause vasodilatation resulting in leakage. These channels are only found in choroidal vasculature. With the use of mineralocorticoid antagonists, down regulation of KCa2.3 channels lead to a reversal of choroidal vessel dilatation and leakage [3]. Figure 1.

As a result, several studies have come to light based on this hypothetical pathogenesis. Orientation of research with the use of mineralocorticoid antagonists has increased, as well as other alternative therapy such as beta-blockers, rifampin, methotrexate, mifepristone ketoconazole, finasteride and aspirin.

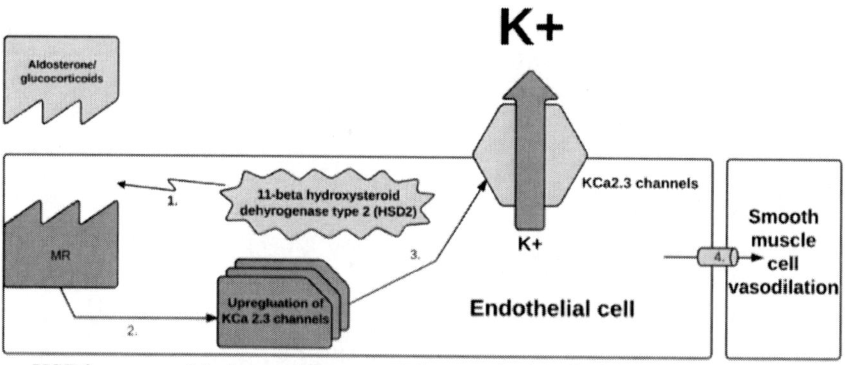

HSD2 enzyme binds to aldosterone/glucocorticoids limiting MR's response (1). MR stimulation induced upregulation of KCa 2.3 channels (2). Membrane bound KCa 2.3 channels release intracellular potassium leading to cellular hyperpolarization (3). Due to electric coupling, the myoedothelial gap junction hyperpolarizes the smooth muscle cell leading to vasodilatation (4).

Figure 1. KCa2.3 channel up regulation and effects.

ALTERNATIVE SYSTEMIC TREATMENTS

Beta-Blockers

Correlation between CSC and obstructive sleep apnea (OSA) has suggested an increase in catecholamines could be a possible etiology [5]. OSA is characterized by increased serum levels of epinephrine and norepinephrine, which may be a risk factor for inducing CSC [6]. Catecholamines, may affect the retinal pigment epithelium (RPE) by changing cyclic adenosine monophosphate (cAMP) concentrations, causing alterations in electrical activity [7]. It has also been shown to induce apoptosis in RPE cells *in vitro* [8]. The use of beta-blockers has been proposed as possible alternative treatment. Previous reports have tried this alternative, however results have been mixed [9].

Beta-blocker, metipranolol was used for acute cases of CSC by Chrapek et al. [10]. The purpose of the investigation was to evaluate the efficiency of administering metipranolol, a non-selective beta-adrenoceptor blocking agent mainly used in ophthalmic solutions to treat patients with ocular hypertension or open-angle glaucoma [11] on newly diagnosed CSC cases.

The double-blind study involved 48 patients with acute CSC. The intervention group was treated with 10 mg of oral metipranolol twice a day.

Metipranolol was prepared by the institution's local pharmacy in oral capsules since no commercial oral formulation exists. Patients were instructed to take the drug until reattachment of neuroepithelium was documented by the research team. Treatment in the metipranolol group ranged from 1 week to 42 weeks for neuroepithelial reattachment while in the placebo group sham treatment ranged from 4 weeks to 48 weeks. The average duration of the detachments in the metipranolol/placebo group was 13 and 12 weeks respectively. In this series, treatment with metipranolol was not statistically significant in reducing the duration of serous detachment of the neuroepithelium in patients with acute onset of CSC.

Although studies testing the use of beta-blockers are scarce, a case report by Tatham and Macfarlane [9] tested a trial of 40 mg twice a day of oral propranolol in two patients with non-resolving or recurrent CSC. Both patients experienced improvement in visual acuity, symptoms and decrease in retinal thickness.

Beta-blockers were one of the first systemic agents to be studied for chronic CSR, but research in this group of drugs was left aside due to other more promising emerging therapies; further testing and new designs in the studies with different beta-blockers is required to clarify the mixed results presented in the published trials.

Eplerenone and Spironolactone

Both drugs have been used by several studies due to their mineralocorticoid antagonism effect. These mineralocorticoid antagonisms are widely used to treat heart failure and hypertension [12]. Spirolactone is an effective aldosterone receptor antagonist but has steroid-related side effects that limit its tolerability. It is also associated with antiandrogenic effects due to the similarity of its structural elements to progesterone [13]. Eplerenone in the other hand, is a spironolactone derivative selective to MR causing insignificant sex related side effects [14]. As a result of its high tolerability, eplerenone is the drug of choice in most studies. Both eplerenone and spirolactone may increase serum potassium levels and are contraindicated in patients with renal insufficiency or significant impairment of renal excretory function [15].

A pilot study by Bousquet et al. [16], treated 13 patients presenting non-regressing CSC for more than 4 months. Patients were treated with 25 mg/day of oral eplerenone for a standard time period of 1 week followed by 50 mg/day for 3 months. The chosen dose of 50 mg/day was used because this is the lowest efficient concentration [14]. After 3 months of medication, central macular thickness and subretinal fluid decreased significantly and visual acuity improved. Central macular thickness decreased from 352 ± 139 μm at baseline to 246 ± 113 μm and 189 ± 99 μm after 1 and 3 months respectively. Subretinal fluid decreased from 175 ± 123 μm to 36 ±55 μm after 3 months. Three patients achieved complete resolution at one month of treatment. BCVA at baseline was 0.52 ± 0.24 and improved to 0.27 ± 0.19 after 3 months.

Following this study, Bousquet et al. [17] carried out a randomized controlled crossover study. Sixteen patients were enrolled with CSC with persistent subretinal fluid for at least 3 months. The treatment consisted of either 50 mg of spironolactone or a placebo per day for 30 days. After treatment, a washout period of 1 week followed by a cross to either spirononolactone or placebo for another 30 days. Treatment sequences were either treatment/placebo (TP) or placebo/treatment (PT).

Statistically significant reduction of SRF in spironolactone treated eyes compared to the same eyes under placebo treatment was shown. There was also a significant reduction in subfoveal choroidal thickness in treated eyes compared to placebo; but no significant changes were seen with the BCVA.

A one-year pilot study by Ghadiali Q et al. [18], patients with chronic CSC characterized by persistent detachment or RPE degeneration were treated with either eplerenone or spirolactone. Acute occurrences of subretinal fluid were also included in the study.

A total of 23 eyes of 14 patients were treated with either 50 mg of spironolactone, eplerenone or both for 12 months. Each patient had the option to switch to the other drug based on side effects, treatment response, or at the discretion of the primary investigator. Patients were initiated with spirolactone principally by its accessibility since this is a generic drug. The majority of patients at the end of the study were treated with spirolactone alone (7/14) as compared with eplerenone (2/14) while a minority of patients were switched medication during treatment (5/14).

The study concluded an improvement in visual acuity and a decrease in subretinal fluid, nonetheless the choroid and macular thickness were not affected. Mean difference in choroidal thickness from baseline was 51.429 μm after 1 month and 37.647 μm and 20.400 μm after six and twelve months respectively which showed no statistical significance. Mean difference in central macular thickness from baseline was 0.200 μm after 1 month interval and 2.810 μm and 31.000 μm after six and twelve months respectively without statistical significance. Mean difference in visual acuity from baseline in the other hand presented statistical significance after twelve months of treatment.

A subgroup for eyes exhibiting subretinal fluid or exudative CSC was evaluated from the 23 patients treated. No significant change was found in central macular thickness, choroidal thickness or BCVA. Subretinal fluid showed statistical significance in subretinal fluid after 6 months and 12 months.

Another pilot study by Singh et al. [19], treated a cohort of 13 patients with chronic CSCR with either 25 mgs or 50 mgs/day of eplerenone with time varied of treatment based on the outcome. The treatment ranged from 38 to 300 days.

The study demonstrated statistical significance in reductions of both horizontal and vertical subretinal fluid measurements. Central subfield thickness along with visual acuity also showed improvement. Mean maximum subretinal fluid height decreased from 131.5 μm at baseline to 15.3 μm at day 181+. Subretinal fluid diameter decreased from average of 2174.4 μm at baseline to 46.9 μm at day 181+. LogMAR visual acuity improved from 0.42 at baseline to 0.29 at day 181+. Central subfield thickness decreased from 339.5 μm at baseline to 270.3 μm at day 181+.

The clinical response to oral mineralocorticoid antagonists has shown promising results in reversing choroidal vasculopathy; but like most of these treatments, it does not escape from publications with opposite results. Hence, further investigation is required to elucidate this inconsistency and determine the optimal treatment dose, duration and to evaluate long-term effects and efficacy.

Methotrexate

Methotrexate (MTX), an antimetabolic drug used in a variety of cases, ranging from cancer therapy to rheumatoid arthritis, has been proposed as an alternative treatment for CSC. MTX prevents pyrimidine and purine synthesis, which is fundamental for DNA and RNA production [20]. This drug also inhibits T cell activation causing immunosuppression [21].

In relation to CSC pathogenesis, MTX has a steroid antagonistic effect [22]. Kurup et al. [23], proposed MTX as a beneficial treatment for patients with chronic CSCR due to its intrinsic properties. Low dose therapy was used to avoid acute toxicity. This low-dose methotrexate therapy has substantial toxicity; side effects include elevation of liver transaminase, acute hepatitis, gastrointestinal disturbances such as anorexia, nausea vomiting and diarrhea, myelosuppression and pneumonitis [24]. Factors as age, duration of exposure to MTX and its cumulative dose, hepatitis B or hepatitis C virus infection, diabetes, obesity and alcohol consumption may increase the hepatotoxic effect of this medication [25]. Weekly MTX dosage ranging between 5-10 mgs was given. Eighty-three percent of the eyes treated had total resolution of the subretinal fluid. The average treatment time was 12 weeks and no patient suffered from MTX toxicity. Improvements in visual acuity, ventral macular thickness and total macular volume were reported. Mean BCVA improved from 20/67 at baseline to 20/35 at 8 weeks. Mean central macular thickness improved from 309 μm at baseline to 213 μm at 8 weeks. Mean total macular volume improved from 8.14 to 7.21 mm^3 at 8 weeks.

Kurup et al. [23], concluded that there could be a possible blockage of corticosteroid receptors by MTX causing an adequate function of RPE pump. They also suggested that the increased adenosine levels in tissue caused by this antimetabolic drug might help stimulate RPE pumps.

An interventional and prospective uncontrolled trial by Abrishami et al. [26], also evaluated the effects of oral methotrexate in patients with chronic CSC; 23 eyes of 23 patients presenting chronic symptomatic CSC and persistent subretinal fluid for longer than 3 months were treated with 7.5 mg per week of oral MTX for a period of 12 weeks. The mean BCVA improved from a 20/40 baseline to a 20/30 at the third month and improved further at 6 month follow up to 20/28. Mean CMT decreased from 375 μm at baseline to 278 μm and 265 μm at the third and sixth month. Mean total macular volume decreased from 9.33 mm^3 at baseline to 8.48 and 8.31 mm^3 at the third and sixth month respectively. Subretinal fluid was completely resolved in 62% of the cases treated. No patient suffered MTX toxicity.

Even though there are no prospective randomized studies, current literature supports MTX as an effective alternative; however, more evidence is required due to the fact that the published reports lack of strong scientific rigor.

Mifepristone

Mifepristone, a glucocorticoid antagonist, binds with glucocorticoid receptors rendering the complex inactive [27]. It is also a potent antiprogesterone agent, used as an abortifacient [28]. Mifepristone has been used to treat meningioma, depression, Cushing's disease, uterine leiomyomata, endometriosis, diabetes and obesity [27]. Its side effects range from skin rashes, nausea, dizziness, fatigue, reversible liver transaminase elevation and endometrial hyperplasia.

Due to its GC antagonistic properties, mifepristone has been used as treatment for chronic CSC. Nielsen and Jampol [29] conducted study involving two separate protocols with 200 mgs of oral mifepristone daily for up to 12 weeks.

The two studies differed in design; the first protocol was a randomized, masked, placebo-controlled trial in which subjects could leave if they did not improve at the 4-week evaluation period. The second protocol was an open label treatment trial and patients could leave the study in case adverse events were encountered.

In the first protocol, 8 patients were enrolled, 4 patients received treatment while the other 4 took a placebo. One patient taking mifepristone and three taking placebo left the study before week 12 due to the lack of improvement. Visual acuity improved by one line in the remaining 3 patients who took mifepristone and the one patient on placebo.

In the second protocol, a total of 13 patients were treated. Six of them expressed subjective improvement in one or both eyes at the end of the treatment period. Six patients were found to have a five-letter or equivalent improvement in visual acuity in one or both eyes. Six patients presented improvement in retinal OCT findings with decrease in subretinal fluid and retinal edema.

In conclusion, 8 of the 16 patients treated in both protocols reported improvement in visual acuity. Seven of them reported an improvement of five letters or greater in visual acuity and improvement in OCT findings.

Although the study was limited to a small size of people, it is clear that mifepristone can play a role in improving chronic CSC treatment. It is important to take into consideration that mifepristone's elevated may limit its use for general treatment.

Ketoconazole

Ketoconazole, an imidazole derivative primarily used for antifungal activity used to lower circulating cortisol levels in Cushing's disease and adrenal hyperplasia [30]. This drug inhibits cytochrome P450 enzymes, which reduces cortisol levels significantly. Ketoconazole use has become controversial because it causes severe hepatotoxicity. The incidence of associated hepatotoxicity with the use of ketoconazole has been reported to be

3.6-4.2% [31]. Other side effects include gastrointestinal complaints, adrenal insufficiency, pruritus, intense fatigue and hair loss [32].

Ketoconazole shows promise due to its adrenocorticoid antagonistic effect, unfortunately it had no effect in a pilot study by Golshahi et al. [33]. Patients were treated with 200 mg a day for four weeks. The treated patients showed no statistical differences in anatomical or functional morphology compared to the control group. Golshahi's paper was criticized by Nielsen and Jampol [29]. They indicated that the treatment was too short and that 200 mg a day is a very low dose that does not cause a significant anti glucocorticoid effect.

In response, Meyerle et al. [34] tested oral ketoconazole at an oral dose of 600 mg per day for four weeks. The investigational case series included five patients with chronic CSC. After four weeks of treatment, median best-corrected Snellen visual acuity remained stable at 20/40. On week 8 follow-up, the median remained the same for visual acuity. Median OCT lesion height at baseline was 116 μm and remained constant at 4 weeks. During week 8 follow-up, median lesion height decreased to 42 μm. The median greatest linear dimension behaved like the median lesion height. At baseline it was reported to be at 1668 μm and lowered slightly to 1660 μm at 4 weeks. At week 8, it decreased drastically to 349 μm.

Despite treatment lasting only 4 weeks, decrease in the median lesion height and greatest linear dimension improved by week 8. Meyerle et al. [34] suggest that the drug effect on cortisol suppression could have persisted despite being off treatment or it could be the natural course of the disorder which tends to have remissions and exacerbations. They consider their result as inconclusive due to the small size of the sample, treatment duration being too short and propose that the dosage of ketoconazole required for optimal antiglucocorticoid effect may need to be increased.

Rifampin

Rifampin, also known as rifampicin is an antibiotic used for the treatment of tuberculosis and leprosy. Its primary mechanism of action is the inhibition of DNA dependent RNA polymerase [35]. Rifampin is usually taken in combination with pyrazinamide, isoniazid and/or ethambutol as antitubercular treatment. Hepatotoxicity is a well-known side effect although it has been shown to have a lower level of liver injury when used in isolation [36]. Rifampicin is a potent inducer of cytochrome P450 3A4, altering glucocorticoid metabolism [37]. This effect causes accelerated steroid metabolism leading to a decrease in steroid serum levels. Due to such alteration in metabolism it has been postulated for the use of CSC.

Shulman et al. [38], concluded oral rifampicin may be a therapeutic option for chronic CSC. They treated twelve patients with 300 mg of oral rifampicin twice per day for at least 3 months.

Mean CMT at baseline was 350 μm improving to 278 μm at the third month. Mean choroidal thickness at presentation was 476 μm and was reduced to 427 μm however improvement wasn't significant. Mean best-corrected visual acuity improved (BCVA) from 20/60 at presentation to a mean of 20/50. Sixty-four percent of the fourteen treated eyes had reduction of subretinal and 42.8% had complete resolution at month 3 of treatment.

The authors of this chapter have limited experience using rifampin as treatment with good results. The availability of rifampin as an anti tubercular agent is easy to obtain in Latin America, this fact associated to administrative issues such as health registration regulation make other local treatments like verteporfin out of range in our country, hence rifampin is a considerable option for selected cases.

We gathered a total of five patients with diagnosis of chronic CSR, all of them had more than 3 months of persistent subretinal fluid and fluorescein angiography showing a subfoveal leaking point, for different reasons they were not able to be treated with other options and rifampin regimen was used. They where treated with 300 mg twice a day for a variable period of time, range from 2 to 10 weeks and hepatic function along with coagulation function tests were performed prior to initiating therapy and every 4 weeks, all of the 5 patients achieved a complete resolution of subretinal fluid and vision improvement. There were no adverse effects of the systemic rifampin in this small group and none of the five patients demonstrated alterations in the laboratory blood tests. (Unpublished data) Figure 2.

Although rifampin displays a promising alternative treatment for CSC, there is a downside with its serious potential risks and this must be taken into account and weighed against its benefits.

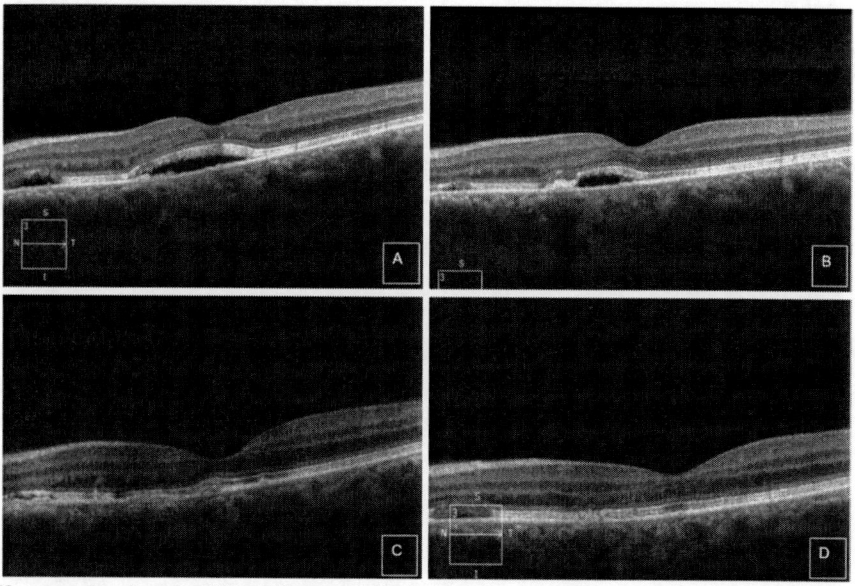

53 yo, male, chronic CSR. Rifampin 600 mg/day for 3 weeks. A) Feb 4, 2014. BCVA 20/30. B) Feb 25, 2014. C) Mar 25, 2014. D) May 6, 2014. BCVA 20/25. Images courtesy of Teodoro Evans MD.

Figure 2. OCT of treated patient with rifampin.

Melatonin

Melatonin is a hormone produced primarily by the pineal gland. It helps regulation of other hormones of the body and plays a role in the body's circadian sleep cycle. Production of melatonin starts at night regardless of behavioral distribution of activity and rest [39]. High production is maintained during the dark phase of the light/dark cycle but is suppressed with light exposure [40]. Involvement in immune system enhancement [41], regulation of GLUT4 expression [39] and anti-angiogenic [42] properties have been described. Melatonin is also thought to down regulate glucocorticoid expression [43, 44], which is why it has been used as an alternative for CSC treatment. The retina synthesizes melatonin is speculated to have a modulatory and protective effect on the retinal pigment epithelial cells, photoreceptors and ganglion cells [45].

Gramajo et al. [46] tested melatonin's efficacy on chronic CSC in a prospective comparative case series. Inclusion criteria were defined as chronic, relapsing CSC with persistent detachments for more than 6 months or chronic recurrent acute detachments with retinal pigment epithelial involvement. Patients with any prior anti-VEGF or laser therapy in the past 3 months, suspicion of choroidal neovascularization, and history of vitrectomy or concomitant ocular conditions were excluded.

A total of 13 patients were treated; 8 patients with 3 mg of oral melatonin three times a day for one month. The five remaining patients were treated with sugar pills and served as a control. At 1-month follow up, 7 of the 8 treated patients showed a significant improvement in BCVA from 0.29 to 0.12. Central macular thickness was significantly reduced in all the treated patients with three patients resulting in complete resolution of subretinal fluid. The control group demonstrated no change in BCVA or CMT. No patient present adverse effects from medication.

There are some key points about the use of melatonin as treatment that justify clinical trials and research. Melatonin is cheap and has an exceptional safety profile with no potential dangerous side effects; such characteristics make it an ideal alternative for treatment. Nonetheless, further investigation and longer follow up is required to prove its adequacy.

Finasteride

An important well demonstrated risk factor for CSC is male gender. The reason as to why male gender is a risk factor is not clear. The tendency of CSC to affect more males than females and to decrease with age correlates with the hormonal behavior. Plasma testosterone levels decrease with age [47]. Therefore it is likely that androgenic effects may play a role in development of CSC.

Finasteride acts by inhibiting 5-alpha reductase causing inhibition of the conversion of testosterone to dihydrotestosterone (DHT). DHT acts as a primary androgen in prostate and hair follicles, which is why finasteride is used for androgenetic alopecia, hirsutism, prostatic hyperplasia and prostate cancer [48, 49]. Adverse effects of this medication are mainly sexual related problems such as erectile dysfunction being the most common followed by ejaculatory dysfunction and loss of libido [49].

Forooghian et al. [50], carried out a pilot study with five patients with chronic CSC. Patients were treated with 5 mg per day of oral finasteride for 3 months. After three months of treatment, medication was withheld for 3 months to observe the outcome. In case BCVA, center-subfield thickness or subretinal volume returned to baseline, patients were allowed to resume finasteride treatment.

Five eyes of five patients were treated. BCVA remained unchanged with no appreciable improvement or worsening while center-subfield macular thickness and subretinal fluid volume declined to its lowest point at the 3-month check up. At the 6-month follow-up both parameters increased slightly but remained lower when compared to baseline levels. Visual acuity and OCT outcomes showed no statistical significance while subretinal fluid volume did.

After discontinuation of treatment, four patients experienced reaccumulation of subretinal fluid. Three of these patients were retreated with finasteride because subretinal fluid volume returned to baseline. Following retreatment all patients experienced subretinal fluid volume decreases.

Androgen receptors have been found in RPE cells and choroid [51, 52]. Although the role androgens play is not known in ocular tissue, hypothesizes suggest that DHT levels might be stimulating choroid androgen receptors and promoting choroid increase in permeability. Due to the potential side effects finasteride can cause, medication adherence is a plausible limitation to this drug as a possible alternative treatment.

Aspirin

Plasminogen activator inhibitor 1 (PAI-1), a major antifibrinolytic agent has been found to be increased in patients with CSC [53]. PAI-1 is the main inhibitor of plasminogen activators such as tissue-type plasminogen activator and urokinase-type plasminogen activator [54]. Risk factors for CSC such as hypertension, sleep disturbances, steroid use and type A behavior are states in which hypercoagulability and platelet aggregation is increased. Studies have suggested the cause of CSC is decreased choroidal blood flow due to increased hypercoagulability and platelet aggregation [55]. Aspirin inhibits arachidonic acid induced platelet aggregation and lowers plasma levels of PAI-1.

Due to aspirin's ability to lower PAI-1 serum levels and inhibit platelet aggregation, Caccavale et al. [56] evaluated the effectiveness of low dose aspirin in treating CSC. The study consisted of treating patients with active or multifocal CSC. Patients were given 100 mg of oral aspiring daily for one month followed by 100 mg on alternate days for five months. Treated subjects were labeled as group A while group B was a control group consisting of patients who had been observed in the same institution. These patients fulfilled the same inclusion and exclusion criteria as group A.

Group A consisted of 109 patients with a mean BCVA of 0.29 ± 0.16 (logMAR) at initial visit while group B had a better mean BCVA of 0.19 ± 0.12. At 1 and 3 months, both groups improved but group A showed greater improvement with 0.14 ± 0.20 and 0.08 ± 0.16 respectively versus 0.21 ± 0.11 and 0.13 ± 0.12 in group B. Patients in group A showed a better and faster recovery. At 6 months, both groups presented similar BVCA with no statistical significance. At the one year and two year follow up, BCVA in group A was better than group B. Group A had a mean BVCA at one year of 0.09 ± 0.17 while group B had a 0.16 ± 0.13. On the two year follow up group A had a BCVA of 0.07 ± 0.13 versus a 0.17 ± 0.13 in group B.

Eighty-six percent of patients in group A experienced no recurrences during follow-up while patients in group B were 57% recurrence free.

Treatment with a low dose of aspirin resulted in a more rapid recovery of visual acuity with fewer recurrences compared to the untreated control group. Limitations to this study include the lack of OCT measured dimensions to see the potential effect it has on anatomical morphology of the retina and choroid. Further investigation is required to prove effectiveness of aspiring in treating CSC.

Helicobacter Pylori Treatment

A correlation between CSC and Helicobacter pylori (H. pylori) has been demonstrated in several studies [57, 58, 59, 60, 61]. H. pylori is a gram-negative bacillus typically found in the stomach associated with gastrointestinal pathologies such as peptic ulcer disease, gastric ulcers, mucosa-associated lymphoid tissue lymphoma and gastric cancer [62]. Immune-mediated damage to choroidal vasculature due to molecular mimicry between antigens expressed by the bacterium and host proteins has been proposed as a possible mechanism in the pathophysiology of this disease [58].

Several studies have tested the use of anti-H. pylori treatment regimen as an alternative treatment for patients with CSC and H. pylori infections with mixed results.

Dang et al. [63] evaluated 53 patients with acute CSC who had tested positive for H. pylori. Twenty-seven patients were treated with 20 mg of omeprazole, 500 mg of clarithromycin and 1 gram of amoxicillin orally, twice a day for 14 days while the remaining 26 patients received placebo treatment. No statistical significance was observed between the two groups, neither the BCVA improved nor the subretinal fluid.

Another study by Barbante Casella et al. [64], treated seventeen patients diagnosed with CSC. Fourteen of the 17 patients were diagnosed with H. pylori infection. All patients were treated with a combination of 500 mg of clarithromycin, 1 gr of amoxicillin and 30 mg of lansoprazole twice a day for seven days. Statistical significance was only shown in BCVA.

A randomized case controlled trial study by Rahbani-Nobar et al. [65] evaluated 58 patients with CSC. Among these patients, 25 were infected with H. pylori while the non-infected severed as a control group. The infected with H. pylori were treated with 500 mg of metronidazole and amoxicillin three times a day for two weeks and omeprazole once daily for 6 weeks. The remaining 25 patients with only CSC received no medication.

The mean subretinal fluid in the treated group was 305.45 ± 161.48 μm and 290 ± 164.38 μm at baseline but failed to show statistical significance in the follow up visits. The subretinal fluid reabsorption time was 9.28 ± 3.2 weeks in the treated group while 11.63 ± 3.18 weeks in the control group did show statistical significance. At baseline the mean visual acuity was 0.10 ± 0.05 (logMAR) in the treated group and 0.09 ± 0.05 in the control group. Sixteen weeks later mean VA improved to 0.003 ± 0.01 in the treated group and 0.004 ± 0.02 in the control group. Both groups showed improvement but the difference did not show statistical significance.

Results have been mixed, however it can be concluded that H. pylori maybe a possible risk factor for the development of CSC. Due to the multifactorial causes of CSC, the possibility of spontaneous regression could have played a big role in patients treated with H. pylori. Given the high prevalence of infections by H. pylori worldwide, incidence of CSC are expected to be a lot higher. After reviewing the published data and the contradictory conclusions of the studies, it is clear that further investigation is required in this field.

CONCLUSION

There is always a predilection among the physicians to give a conservative approach to acute CSC due to the high rate of spontaneous healing. The main purpose is to educate and inform the patient to continue control in case therapy should be required. In case, the disease were to become chronic and recalcitrant a necessity to intervene may be required. Ideally local therapy in chronic CSR is the primary choice due to the possible systemic effects oral drugs could have on the patient. The use of systemic therapy for chronic CSR is not a common practice, and it is mainly limited as a last resource to those cases in which other modalities such as conventional laser, micropulse laser or photodynamic therapy with verteporfin are not available or by some reason are contraindicated.

So far, promising results can be achieved with some of the previously described therapies. Although most of these publications propose non-conventional options, most of these studies investigate on a small number of patients with short follow-ups. Larger number of cases and randomized studies need to be published to get conclusive data about long-term efficacy, recurrences, safety and tolerance. Most results seen are mixed and sometimes inconsistent leading to limitation in clinical use. Guidelines to establish protocols are required but due to current results it can be arduous. More studies are recommended to reach consent and to establish these different modalities of treatment. The lack of treatment options for CSC has been an initiative to institutions in which research is closer to understanding the underlying cause of this condition. A greater acknowledgment of the mechanics of this disease will improve the therapeutic strategy ophthalmologists take.

References

[1] Iacono P, Battaglia Parodi M, Falcomatà B, Bandello F. Central Serous Chorioretinopathy Treatments: A Mini Review. *Ophthalmic Res.* 2015; 55(2):76-83. doi:10.1159/000441502.

[2] Kitzmann AS, Pulido JS, Diehl NN, Hodge DO, Burke JP. The Incidence of Central Serous Chorioretinopathy in Olmsted County, Minnesota, 1980-2002. *Ophthalmology.* 2008;115(1):169-173. doi:10.1016/j.ophtha.2007.02.032.

[3] Zhao M, Célérier I, Bousquet E et al. Mineralocorticoid receptor is involved in rat and human ocular chorioretinopathy. *J. Clin. Invest.* 2012;122(7):1-8. doi:10.1172/JCI61427DS1.

[4] Wilkinson-Berka JL, Tan G, Jaworski K, Miller AG. Identification of a retinal aldosterone system and the protective effects of mineralocorticoid receptor antagonism on retinal vascular pathology. *Circ. Res.* 2009;104 (1):124-133. doi:10.1161/CIRCRESAHA.108.176008.

[5] Yavas GF, Kusbeci T, Kasikci M et al. Obstructive sleep apnea in patients with central serous chorioretinopathy. *Curr. Eye Res.* 2014;39 (1):88-92. doi:10.3109/02713683.2013.824986.

[6] Leveque TK, Yu L, Musch DC, Chervin RD, Zacks DN. Central serous chorioretinopathy and risk for obstructive sleep apnea. *Sleep Breath.* 2007;11(4):253-257. doi:10.1007/s11325-007-0112-3.

[7] Frambach DA, Fain GL, Farber DB, Bok D. Beta adrenergic receptors on cultured human retinal pigment epithelium. *Invest. Ophthalmol. Vis. Sci.* 1990;31(9):1767-1772. http://www.ncbi.nlm.nih.gov/entrez/query.fcgi?cmd=Retrieve&db=PubMed&dopt=Citation&list_uids=2170293.

[8] Sibayan SA, Kobuch K, Spiegel D et al. Epinephrine, but not dexamethasone, induces apoptosis in retinal pigment epithelium cells *in vitro*: possible implications on the pathogenesis of central serous chorioretinopathy. *Graefe's Arch. Clin. Exp. Ophthalmol.* 2000;238(6): 515-519. http://www.ncbi.nlm.nih.gov/pubmed/10943677.

[9] Tatham A, Macfarlane A. The use of propranolol to treat central serous chorioretinopathy: an evaluation by serial OCT. *J. Ocul. Pharmacol. Ther.* 2006;22(2):145-149. doi:10.1089/jop.2006.22.145.

[10] Chrapek O, Jirkova B, Kandrnal V, Rehak J, Sin M. Treatment of central serous chorioretinopathy with beta-blocker metipranolol. *Biomed. Pap. Med. Fac. Univ. Palacky Olomouc Czech Repub.* 2013;159(1):3-6.

[11] Battershill PE, Sorkin EM. Ocular Metipranolol. *Drugs.* 1988;36(5):601-615. doi:10.2165/00003495-198836050-00004.

[12] Struthers A, Krum H, Williams GH. A comparison of the aldosterone-blocking agents eplerenone and spironolactone. *Clin. Cardiol.* 2008;31 (4):153-158. doi:10.1002/clc.20324.

[13] de Gasparo M, Joss U, Ramjoué HP et al. Three new epoxy-spirolactone derivatives: characterization *in vivo* and *in vitro*. *J. Pharmacol. Exp. Ther.* 1987;240(2):650-656. http://www.ncbi.nlm.nih.gov/pubmed/2949071.

[14] Pitt B, Remme W, Zannad F et al. Eplerenone, a selective aldosterone blocker, in patients with left ventricular dysfunction after myocardial infarction. *N. Engl. J. Med.* 2003;348(14):1309-1321. doi:10.1056/NEJMoa030207.

[15] Weinberger MH, Roniker B, Krause SL, Weiss RJ. Eplerenone, a Selective Aldosterone Blocker, in mild-to-moderate hypertension. *Am. J. Hypertens.* 2002;15(8):709-716. doi:10.1016/S0895-7061(02)02957-6.

[16] Bousquet E, Beydoun T, Zhao M, Hassan L, Offret O, Behar-Cohen F. Mineralocorticoid receptor antagonism in the treatment of chronic central serous chorioretinopathy: a pilot study. *Retina.* 2013;33(10): 2096-2102. doi:10.1097/IAE.0b013e318297a07a.

[17] Bousquet E, Beydoun T, Rothschild P-R et al. Spironolactone for Nonresolving Central Serous Chorioretinopathy: a Randomized Controlled Crossover Study. *Retina*. 2015;35(12):2505-2515. doi:10.1097/IAE.0000000000000614.

[18] Ghadiali Q, Jung JJ, Yu S, Patel SN, Yannuzzi LA. Central Serous Chorioretinopathy Treated With Mineralocorticoid Antagonists: a One-Year Pilot Study. *Retina*. 2015:611-618. doi:10.1097/IAE.0000000000000748.

[19] Singh RP, Sears JE, Bedi R, Schachat AP, Ehlers JP, Kaiser PK. Oral eplerenone for the management of chronic central serous chorioretinopathy. *Int. J. Ophthalmol*. 2015;8(2):310-314. doi:10.3980/j.issn.2222-3959.2015.02.17.

[20] Whittle SL, Hughes RA. Folate supplementation and methotrexate treatment in rheumatoid arthritis: A review. *Rheumatology*. 2004;43(3):267-271. doi:10.1093/rheumatology/keh088.

[21] Strauss G, Osen W, Debatin K-M. Induction of apoptosis and modulation of activation and effector function in T cells by immunosuppressive drugs. *Clin. Exp. Immunol*. 2002;128(2):255-266. doi:1777 [pii].

[22] Wessels JAM, Huizinga TWJ, Guchelaar H-J. Recent insights in the pharmacological actions of methotrexate in the treatment of rheumatoid arthritis. *Rheumatol*. 2008;47 (3):249-255. doi:10.1093/rheumatology/kem279.

[23] Kurup S, Oliver A, Emanuelli A, Hau V, Callanan D. Low-dose methotrexate for the treatment of chronic central serous chorioretinopathy: A Retrospective Analysis. *Retina*. 2012;32(10):2096-2101. http://0-ovidsp.ovid.com.wam.city.ac.uk/ovidweb.cgi?T=JS&PAGE=reference&D=ovftn&NEWS=N&AN=00006982-201211000-00015.

[24] Gutierrez-Ureña S, Molina JF, García CO, Cuéllar ML, Espinoza LR. Pancytopenia secondary to methotrexate therapy in rheumatoid arthritis. *Arthritis Rheum*. 1996;39(2):272-276. http://www.ncbi.nlm.nih.gov/pubmed/10063319.

[25] Sotoudehmanesh R, Anvari B, Akhlaghi M, Shahraeeni S, Kolahdoozan S. Methotrexate hepatotoxicity in patients with rheumatoid arthritis. *Middle East J. Dig. Dis*. 2010;2(2):104-109. http://www.pubmedcentral.nih.gov/articlerender.fcgi?artid=4154822&tool=pmcentrez&rendertype=abstract.

[26] Abrishami M, Mousavi M, Hosseini S-M, Norouzpour A. Treatment of Chronic Central Serous Chorioretinopathy with Oral Methotrexate. *J. Ocul. Pharmacol. Ther.* 2015;31(8):468-475. doi:10.1089/jop.2014.0173.

[27] Cadepond F, Ulmann A, Baulieu EE. RU486 (mifepristone): mechanisms of action and clinical uses. *Annu. Rev. Med.* 1997;48:129-156. doi:10.1146/annurev.med.48.1.129.

[28] Allen R, O'Brien BM. Uses of misoprostol in obstetrics and gynecology. *Rev. Obstet. Gynecol.* 2009;2(3):159-168. doi:10.3909/riog0055.

[29] Nielsen JS, Jampol LM. Oral mifepristone for chronic central serous chorioretinopathy. *Retina.* 2011;31(9):1928-1936. doi:10.1097/IAE.0b013e31821c3ef6.

[30] Comte-Perret S, Zanchi A, Gomez F. Long-term low-dose ketoconazole treatment in bilateral macronodular adrenal hyperplasia. *Endocrinol. diabetes Metab. case reports.* 2014;2014(December):140083. doi:10.1530/EDM-14-0083.

[31] Yan JY, Nie XL, Tao QM, Zhan SY, Zhang Y De. Ketoconazole associated hepatotoxicity: a systematic review and meta-analysis. *Biomed. Environ. Sci.* 2013;26(7):605-610. doi:10.3967/0895-3988.2013.07.013.

[32] Castinetti F, Guignat L, Giraud P et al. Ketoconazole in cushing's disease: Is it worth a try. *J. Clin. Endocrinol. Metab.* 2014;99(5):1623-1630. doi:10.1210/jc.2013-3628.

[33] Golshahi A, Klingmüller D, Holz FG, Eter N. Ketoconazole in the treatment of central serous chorioretinopathy: A pilot study. *Acta Ophthalmol.* 2010;88(5):576-581. doi:10.1111/j.1755-3768.2008.01467.x.

[34] Meyerle CB, Freund KB, Bhatnagar P, Shah V, Yannuzzi L a. Ketoconazole in the treatment of chronic idiopathic central serous chorioretinopathy. *Retina.* 2007;27(7):943-946. doi:10.1097/IAE.0b013e318050ca69.

[35] Campbell E a. EA, Korzheva N, Mustaev A et al. Structural mechanism for rifampicin inhibition of bacterial rna polymerase. *Cell.* 2001;104(6):901-912. doi:10.1016/S0092-8674(01)00286-0.

[36] Menzies D, Long R, Trajman A et al. Adverse events with 4 months of rifampin therapy or 9 months of isoniazid therapy for latent tuberculosis infection: A randomized trial. *Ann. Intern. Med.* 2008;149(10):689-697. doi:149/10/689 [pii].

[37] McAllister WA, Thompson PJ, Al-Habet SM, Rogers HJ. Rifampicin reduces effectiveness and bioavailability of prednisolone. *Br. Med. J.* 1983;286(6369):923-925. doi:10.1136/bmj.286.6369.923.

[38] Shulman S, Goldenberg D, Schwartz R et al. Oral Rifampin treatment for longstanding chronic central serous chorioretinopathy. *Graefe's Arch. Clin. Exp. Ophthalmol.* 2016;254(1):15-22. doi:10.1007/s00417-015-2989-z.

[39] Cipolla-Neto J, Amaral FG, Afeche SC, Tan DX, Reiter RJ. Melatonin, energy metabolism, and obesity: A review. *J. Pineal Res.* 2014;56(4): 371-381. doi:10.1111/jpi.12137.

[40] Lockley SW, Brainard GC, Czeisler CA. High sensitivity of the human circadian melatonin rhythm to resetting by short wavelength light. *J. Clin. Endocrinol. Metab.* 2003;88(9):4502-4505. doi:10.1210/jc.2003-030570.

[41] Nelson RJ, Drazen DL. Melatonin mediates seasonal adjustments in immune function. *Reprod. Nutr. Dev.* 1999;39(3):383-398. doi:S092652 8799800641 [pii].

[42] Lissoni P, Rovelli F, Malugani F, Bucovec R, Conti A, Maestroni GJ. Anti-angiogenic activity of melatonin in advanced cancer patients. *Neuro Endocrinol. Lett.* 2001;22(1):45-47. http://www.ncbi.nlm.nih.gov/ pubmed/11335879.

[43] Gupta S, Haldar C. Physiological crosstalk between melatonin and glucocorticoid receptor modulates T-cell mediated immune responses in a wild tropical rodent, Funambulus pennanti. *J. Steroid Biochem. Mol. Biol.* 2013;134(1):23-36. doi:10.1016/j.jsbmb.2012.09.013.

[44] Asainz Rm, Mayo Jc, Reiter Rj, Antolin I, Esteban Mm, Rodriguez C. Melatonin Regulates Glucocorticoid Receptor: An Answer to its antiapoptotic action in thymus. *Faseb J.* 1999;13(12):1547-1556. http:// www.fasebj.org/content/13/12/1547.full.

[45] Tosini G, Baba K, Hwang CK, Iuvone PM. Melatonin: An underappreciated player in retinal physiology and pathophysiology. *Exp. Eye Res.* 2012;103:82-89. doi:10.1016/j.exer.2012.08.009.

[46] Gramajo AL, Marquez GE, Torres VE, Juarez CP, Rosenstein RE, Luna JD. Therapeutic benefit of melatonin in refractory central serous chorioretinopathy. *Eye (Lond).* 2015;29(8):1036-1045. doi:10.1038/eye. 2015.104.

[47] Stanworth RD, Jones TH. Testosterone for the aging male; current evidence and recommended practice. *Clin. Interv. Aging.* 2008;3(1):25-44.

[48] Townsend KA, Marlowe KF. Relative safety and efficacy of finasteride for treatment of hirsutism. *Ann. Pharmacother.* 2004;38(6):1070-1073. doi:10.1345/aph.1D461.

[49] Mysore V. Finasteride and sexual side effects. *Indian Dermatol. Online J.* 2012;3(1):62-65. doi:10.4103/2229-5178.93496.

[50] Forooghian F, Meleth A, D MD MS et al. Finasteride for Chronic Central Serous Chorioretinopathy. *Retina.* 2011;31(4):766-771. doi:10. 1097/IAE.0b013e3181f04a35.

[51] Rocha EM, Wickham L a, da Silveira L a et al. Identification of androgen receptor protein and 5alpha-reductase mRNA in human ocular tissues. *Br. J. Ophthalmol.* 2000;84(1):76-84. doi:10.1136/bjo.84.1.76.

[52] Fuchsjäger-Mayrl G, Nepp J, Schneeberger C et al. Identification of estrogen and progesterone receptor mRNA expression in the conjunctiva of premenopausal women. *Invest. Ophthalmol. Vis. Sci.* 2002;43(9): 2841-2844.

[53] Iijima H, Iida T, Murayama K, Imai M, Gohdo T. Plasminogen activator inhibitor 1 in central serous chorioretinopathy. *Am. J. Ophthalmol.* 1999;127(4):477-478. doi:10.1016/S0002-9394(98)00378-X.

[54] Yasar Yildiz S, Kuru P, Toksoy Oner E, Agirbasli M. Functional stability of plasminogen activator inhibitor-1. *Sci. World J.* 2014;2014. doi:10.1155/2014/858293.

[55] Kitaya N, Nagaoka T, Hikichi T et al. Features of abnormal choroidal circulation in central serous chorioretinopathy. *Br. J. Ophthalmol.* 2003; 87(6):709-712. doi:10.1136/bjo.87.6.709.

[56] Caccavale A, Romanazzi F, Imparato M, Negri A, Morano A, Ferentini F. Low-dose aspirin as treatment for central serous chorioretinopathy. *Clin. Ophthalmol.* 2010;4:899-903. http://www.pubmedcentral.nih.gov/ articlerender.fcgi?artid=2921298&tool=pmcentrez&rendertype=abstract.

[57] Asensio-Sánchez VM, Rodríguez-Delgado B, García-Herrero E, Cabo-Vaquera V, García-Loygorri C. [Central serous chorioretinopathy as an extradigestive manifestation of Helicobacter pylori gastric infection]. *Arch. Soc. Esp. Oftalmol.* 2008;83(3):177-182. http://www.ncbi.nlm.nih. gov/pubmed/18311677.

[58] Giusti C. Association of Helicobacter pylori with central serous chorioretinopathy: Hypotheses regarding pathogenesis. *Med. Hypotheses.* 2004;63(3):524-527. doi:10.1016/j.mehy.2004.02.020.

[59] Cotticelli L, Borrelli M, D'Alessio AC et al. Central serous chorioretinopathy and Helicobacter pylori. *Eur. J. Ophthalmol.* 2006;16 (2):274-278. http://www.ncbi.nlm.nih.gov/pubmed/16703546.

[60] Giusti C. [Central serous chorioretinopathy: a new extragastric manifestation of Helicobacter pylori?: Analysis of a clinical case]. *Clin. Ter*. 2001;152(6):393-397. http://www.ncbi.nlm.nih.gov/pubmed/11865 536.

[61] Misiuk-Hojło M, Michałowska M, Turno-Krecicka A. Helicobacter pylori--a risk factor for the developement of the central serous chorioretinopathy. *Klin. Oczna*. 2009;111(1-3):30-32. http://www.ncbi.nlm.nih.gov/pubmed/19517842.

[62] Elvira Garza-González, Guillermo Ignacio Perez-Perez, Héctor Jesús Maldonado-Garza and FJB-P. A review of Helicobacter pylori diagnosis, treatment, and methods to detect eradication. *World J. Gastroenterol*. 2014;20(6):1438-1449. doi:10.3748/wjg.v20.i6.1438.

[63] Dang Y, Mu Y, Zhao M, Li L, Guo Y, Zhu Y. The effect of eradicating Helicobacter pylori on idiopathic central serous chorioretinopathy patients. *Ther. Clin. Risk Manag*. 2013;9(1):355-360. doi:10.2147/TCRM.S50407.

[64] Marcelo A, Casella B, Fabri Berbel R et al. Helicobacter pylori as a potential target for the treat- ment of central serous chorioretinopathy. *Clinics*. 2012;67(9):1047-1052. doi:10.6061/clinics/2012(09)11.

[65] Rahbani-Nobar MB, Javadzadeh A, Ghojazadeh L, Rafeey M, Ghorbanihaghjo A. The effect of Helicobacter pylori treatment on remission of idiopathic central serous chorioretinopathy. *Mol. Vis*. 2011; 17(January):99-103.

Reviewed by: Carlos Arrea-Baixench. Editorial Committee, Acta Medica Costarricense. San Jose Costa Rica.

RELATED NOVA PUBLICATION

CENTRAL SEROUS CHORIORETINOPATHY AND SLEEP DISORDERS*

Kiersten Pollard, MD, Mingwu Wang, MD, PhD and John Christoforidis†, MD
Department of Ophthalmology and Vision Science,
University of Arizona College of Medicine

A healthy, 34-year-old, African American man presents with complaints of a black spot affecting his left eye's central vision, which appeared acutely, 1 month before presentation. He reports no associated pain, photophobia, diplopia, or flashing lights. Visual acuity is 20/15 in his right eye, $20/20^{-1}$ in his left eye. Ocular examination is significant for a serous retinal detachment in the left eye, measuring about 1 disk diameter, located in the inferotemporal foveal region. Optical coherence tomography (OCT) displays a corresponding neurosensory retinal detachment. Intravenous fluorescein angiography reveals an early phase hyperfluorescent spot in the same area, which gradually enlarges centrifugally through the recirculation phase. The diagnosis of central serous chorioretinopathy (CSC) in the left eye is made.

* The full version of this chapter can be found in *Eye Diseases Associated with Sleep Disorders*, edited by Mingwu Wang, published by Nova Science Publishers, Inc, New York, 2015.

† jchristiforidis@eyes.arizona.edu

BIBLIOGRAPHY

Swept-source optical coherence tomography: a color atlas	
LCCN	2015020370
Type of material	Book
Personal name	Teo, Kelvin Y. C., author.
Main title	Swept-source optical coherence tomography: a color atlas / Kelvin Y.C. Teo, Wong Chee Wai, Andrew S.H. Tsai, Daniel S.W. Ting, Singapore National Eye Centre, Singapore; edited by Lee Shu Yen and Gemmy C.M. Cheung, Singapore National Eye Centre, Singapore; preface by Wong Tien Yin, Singapore National Eye Centre, Singapore.
Published/Produced	Singapore; Hackensack, NJ: World Scientific, 2015.
Description	xii, 56 pages: illustrations (some color); 22 cm
ISBN	9789814704212 (pbk.: alk. paper)
	9814704210 (pbk.: alk. paper)
LC classification	RE551 .T46 2015
Related names	Wong, Chee Wai, author.
	Tsai, Andrew S. H., author.
	Ting, Daniel S. W., author.
	Lee, Shu Yen, editor.
	Cheung, Gemmy C. M., editor.
Contents	Introduction to SS-OCT -- Retinal vascular disease -- Macula disorders -- Central serous chorioretinopathy -- Age related macular degeneration -- Vitreo macular interface disease --

	Myopia -- Inflammatory conditions -- Miscellaneous conditions.
Subjects	Retinal Diseases--diagnosis--Atlases.
	Tomography, Optical Coherence--methods--Atlases.
Notes	Includes index.
Eye diseases associated with sleep disorders	
LCCN	2015939637
Type of material	Book
Main title	Eye diseases associated with sleep disorders / Mingwu Wang, editor.
Published/Created	New York: Nova Biomedical, c2015.
Description	ix, 144 p.: ill. (chiefly col.); 24 cm.
ISBN	9781634828949
	1634828941
LC classification	RE46 .E93 2015
Related names	Wang, Mingwu (Ophthalmologist)
Contents	Sleep disorders and neuroregulation -- Floppy eyelid syndrome and obstructive sleep apnea -- Dry eye disease and sleep deprivation -- Keratoconus and obstructive sleep apnea -- Retinal vein occlusion and obstructive sleep apnea -- Central serous chorioretinopathy and sleep disorders -- Diabetic retinopathy and obstructive sleep apnea -- Glaucoma and sleep disorders -- Papilledema and sleep disorders -- Nonarteritic anterior ischemic optic neuropathy and obstructive sleep apnea.
Subjects	Eye--Diseases.
	Sleep disorders--Complications.
	Eye Diseases--physiopathology.
	Sleep Wake Disorders--complications.
Notes	Includes bibliographical references and index.
Series	Eye and vision research developments
	Eye and vision research developments series.

INDEX

E

F

G

H

I

K

L

T

U

V

W

X